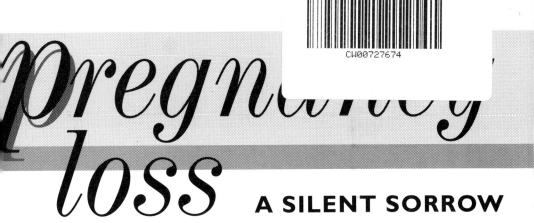

pregnancy loss

A SILENT SORROW

Guidance and support for you and your family

Ingrid Kohn &
Perry-Lynn Moffitt

WITH WELLBEING,
THE HEALTH RESEARCH CHARITY
FOR WOMEN & BABIES

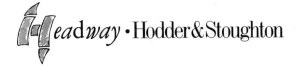

Headway · Hodder & Stoughton

To Miriam and Tova, with love,
I K

To Edward, David, and Justine, with love,
P-L M

A catalogue record for this title is available from the British Library

ISBN 0 340 60644 4

First published in US by Bantam Doubleday Dell Publishing Group, Inc., 1992
First published by Hodder Headline 1994

Impression number   10 9 8 7 6 5 4 3 2 1
Year   1999 1998 1997 1996 1995 1994

Copyright © 1992, 1994, Ingrid Kohn and Perry-Lynn Moffitt

Typeset by Wearset, Boldon, Tyne and Wear.
Printed in Great Britain for Hodder & Stoughton Educational, a division of Hodder Headline Plc, 338 Euston Road, London NW1 3BH by Page Bros (Norwich) Ltd.

CONTENTS

A NOTE FROM THE AUTHORS

We have chosen to refer to women and men who have suffered pregnancy losses as 'mothers' and 'fathers.' This reflects the feelings of many bereaved couples we interviewed that they became mothers and fathers through the love they gave their unborn or newborn children, no matter how briefly they had known them.

We confronted the biases language can convey and have tried to avoid sexist words and concepts. By addressing our readers as 'you' and by referring to each member of a couple as a 'partner' instead of a 'spouse,' 'husband,' or 'wife,' we hoped to encompass all grieving parents, be they female, male, single, married, gay, or heterosexual. We hope we have succeeded and that you will find solace within these pages no matter what your circumstances might be. We have endeavoured to make the book accessible to all people whose lives are touched by pregnancy loss and hope you will feel free to pass this volume along to a friend, relative, or professional who might find it useful.

A *Silent Sorrow* developed a life of its own as we began to conduct our research and interview parents. We had originally planned a separate chapter for single women who, by choice or by chance, found themselves pregnant and then lost their babies. After we interviewed several single women, we discovered that whether or not they had conceived their babies as part of a loving but unmarried couple, or were artificially inseminated, or lived alone much against their will, it made little difference to their experience of the loss. Although some single women admitted to feeling criticized or ostracized for having been pregnant, a topic that is explored in Chapters 10 and 11, most shared the same elements of grief and disappointment as married mothers. We hope single women reading this book will find our approach helpful.

This book was written to provide guidance, comfort, and hope to all parents who have experienced an unwanted pregnancy loss, including those who have ended an impaired pregnancy. We considered using terms such as 'fetus' and 'embryo' when discussing abnormal pregnancies and abortions, realizing this language was more in keeping with a pro-choice stance. In the end, we continued to refer to the 'unborn baby.' We felt compelled to acknowledge this common grief: no matter what the cause of their loss, bereaved parents mourn for someone who was dear to them, someone who was supposed to be their 'baby.' If the words we chose are imperfect, they still represent our sincerest attempt to give expression to this universal sorrow.

INGRID KOHN
San Diego, California

PERRY-LYNN MOFFITT
New York City, New York

FOREWORD

To lose a baby is something most of us do not have to endure. We can try to imagine the pain and anguish involved, but when it gets too unbearable, we can switch off. This is a luxury denied those women and men who do lose a much longed for baby. I have been moved to tears on innumerable occasions, when hearing a woman who has lost a child, either during pregnancy, or at birth, describe the intense grief, guilt, anger or emptiness that she felt, not just at the time, but throughout succeeding years.

The fact that this grief is so enduring was brought home to me when I introduced a Bill, now law, redefining stillbirth, whilst I was a Member of Parliament. I received letters from women all over the country, some in their seventies who were still haunted by their grief all over the country, some in their seventies who were still haunted by their grief and guilt.

In days gone by, many doctors and midwives, with the best of intentions, swept the problem out of the way and cheerily told the mother not to worry, she could have another baby. This often involved the baby being disposed of, unseen, unheld and with no loving farewell.

We know now that this is not the right way to help parents come to terms with the loss of their baby. Parents are encouraged to grieve, to hold and to participate in their baby's funeral. Times change, and what would have been considered morbid is now recognised as essential as part of the grieving process.

Professionals, friends and relatives still have a lot to learn about how to help and how to cope. Fear of saying the wrong thing often leads to an intolerable silence which can cause even more misery.

This book will be invaluable, not just to those mothers and fathers, grandmothers and grandfathers, and other relatives who have to face this tragedy, but also for the many professionals who want to help and comfort but don't know how.

Rosie Barnes
Director, WellBeing
London, April 1994

THE GRIEF OF PREGNANCY LOSS

P arents who endure any form of pregnancy loss share many common issues and concerns. They have all lost the reality of becoming parents or of presenting their other children with a new baby brother or sister, at least temporarily. Yet every loss is suffered individually by each bereaved parent, who must cope with the sorrow at hand and who may have concerns about the future as well.

Pregnancy loss and infant death have been with us since the birth of humankind. However, it has been only in recent years that we have devoted much scholarly study, medical scrutiny, and emotional honesty to this frequent and tragic event. In this book, the term 'pregnancy loss' encompasses the entire spectrum of misfortune during pregnancy, including miscarriage, ectopic pregnancy, losses following medical crises, stillbirth, newborn death, and ending the pregnancy when the baby's life or health is compromised. The term embraces all losses that occur whenever a wanted pregnancy has ended.

This particular section examines the grief you may feel as a mother or father when you suffer a pregnancy loss. By exploring these different responses to pregnancy loss, you can begin to find some solace and the will to face your future again with hope.

CHAPTER I

WHEN AN UNBORN OR NEWBORN BABY DIES

Heather's Story

Mike and I were thrilled about my pregnancy, which was our first. I decided to stop working in the eighth month because I became uncomfortable and tired, but apart from this, I didn't have any problems at all.

A few days after my regular checkup in the last month, we were at the pictures when I felt this violent movement. The next day I didn't feel the baby move all day and finally called Mike at work to tell him. He tried to say that everything was probably okay and normal, but we were anxious for my doctor's appointment, which was the next day, two weeks before my due date.

The nurse tried to hear a heartbeat with a sonicaid and then came in with a stethoscope. She was very matter-of-fact, which I couldn't believe. It seemed like a bad dream that we would awaken from to find the baby okay. Then the doctor came in and couldn't hear a heartbeat either. He said to go to the hospital for a scan, which confirmed that the baby had died.

Mike and I both broke down. Mike kept sobbing 'Why, why?' over and over. The doctor stayed and tried to answer our questions, but mostly we wanted to know why this had happened, and he couldn't answer that right away. He suggested that I go home to wait until labour started naturally.

Three days later, I went into labour. Mike drove me to the hospital, but the nurses on duty hadn't been told why we were there. It was a very awkward situation. Being on the maternity and labour ward where everyone else was giving birth was even worse.

The labour took a long time. The doctor gave me Syntocinon to help, and the pain was terrible. He finally gave me some Pethadine. Then they wheeled me into the delivery room, and our daughter was born. The umbilical cord had wrapped around her neck, which was probably why she had died. She was a perfectly normal-looking baby. I held her in my arms and cried and cried. After carrying her for almost nine months, it just all seemed so senseless. We had picked the name Melinda for her in advance, and we gave her that name.

We decided on cremation and wanted to scatter the ashes in our backyard, where we planted an azalea bush for Melinda. Our vicar and close family came. The day of the funeral, I remember thinking life would never be good again, that this sadness would never end.

For a few months, I thought about the baby all the time. Even after I started to feel better, certain things really upset me, like when a close friend called to tell me she was pregnant. I started crying, but I pulled myself together to say 'congratulations.' It was terrible.

I became pregnant in the autumn. This next pregnancy was a very emotional time. We couldn't enjoy it, or share our joy with family and friends the way I would have liked, because we felt so cautious. We didn't breathe easily until our next baby, Sophie, was born, crying and kicking!

We say a prayer by Melinda's azalea bush every spring. Losing her changed our lives. Mike and I realize how lucky we are to have Sophie. We don't take things so much for granted anymore.

With your pregnancy loss, you probably felt as if your world had turned upside down in the space of a few hours or days. You had expected a new life and instead you were confronted with death. The hopes and plans you had for your future and your baby were wrenched from you.

Now, instead of feeling expectant and special, you may be left with a terrible sense of frustration and even failure. Your life and goals can suddenly feel totally beyond your control. This may be true whether your loss was a miscarriage or a full-term stillbirth, and whether or not the pregnancy had been planned. Any pregnancy loss can turn the love and hopes you had nurtured for your expected baby into grief.

Reminders of your tragedy may be all around you. Friends and relatives may have sent you baby presents and congratulations cards. Perhaps you had moved to a larger home, or set up a room for the baby, and your loss renders all your plans meaningless. You may suddenly find yourself painfully jealous of other expectant couples, even if they are close friends or family. Loved ones who were caring and attentive while you were expecting a baby may suddenly avoid you after your loss, or say things that are well-meaning but that hurt you.

No matter what kind of pregnancy loss you experienced, you are probably unprepared for the pain and anguish you feel. This emotional trauma may take a long time to heal, as you have lost someone who was a real part of you and your hoped-for future.

Grieving for Your Baby

Of all life events, having and raising children are among the most significant. You may have taken for granted from childhood that you would someday have a family of your own. No matter what your career orientation may be, your womanhood or manhood can be powerfully affirmed by bearing or fathering a child. Pregnancy and parenthood are passages into adulthood that bestow a special status on you, within both your family and your community. Pregnancy even represents a chance to overcome mortality, as you contemplate the continuation of your family line.

Pregnancy often establishes a special realtionship between parents and their expected baby. Until recently, popular wisdom held that parents were incapable of caring deeply about their unborn baby because they didn't really know their child. But in the 1970s two American paediatricians, John Kennell and Marshall Klause, showed through their research that parents' emotional attachment, or bonding, begins early in the pregnancy.

Perhaps the baby became real for you the moment the conception was confirmed. As your preganancy progressed, the baby's place in your family may have become more firmly established. You may have wondered whom the baby would look like and imagined your child in your extended family, playing with cousins and grandparents. You may have dreamed about the baby's future, wondering if your child would go into your profession, or attend the same school.

Your attachment to your unborn baby might have been enhanced by medical technology, which allowed you to hear a heartbeat ten to twelve weeks after conception and to see your unborn baby with an ultrasound scan as early as seven or eight weeks into the pregnancy. If you had you may have discovered the baby's sex and may have even named your child quite early in the pregnancy. Experiencing the pregnancy in these ways can have made your unborn child very real and dear to you.

Some ambivalence during pregnancy is common. If your pregnancy was unplanned or you had worried about becoming a parent, you still had a relationship to your child and will probably go through a grieving period. Mourning can be especially difficult under these circumstances, because you may be feeling burdened with guilt as well as sorrow.

In the weeks and months following your loss, you may mourn your baby and the loss of your dreams for a future with that child. Grief can be frightening and overwhelming, especially if you do not realize that it is a natural response to your loss and that, when allowed to run its course, it will eventually be less painful.

If you could step back from your grief, you would see it as a process with different phases or stages that can last many months and change over time. At the moment of your tragedy, you probably felt shock and denial, followed by severe emotional distress, including anxiety and depression. As the grieving process continues, you may experience phases of anger, guilt, and jealousy as well as an overwhelming yearning for your baby.

Some parents develop symptoms of post-traumatic stress syndrome following a pregnancy loss. They respond to their tragedy with the same intense reactions as do victims of extreme physical and emotional traumas such as fires, plane crashes, or rapes. Parents suffering from this disorder may display such disparate symptoms as reliving the events in great detail, or forming a kind of amnesia about the loss of their child.

No matter what form your grief takes, you will eventually sense a gradual lessening of emotional pain as you come to terms with your loss. This final phase of mourning is often referred to as grief resolution or integration.

Mothers and fathers often experience and grieve a pregnancy loss differently. Because the mother physically carries the pregnancy, she usually bonds earlier and more strongly with the baby than the father. When the pregnancy ends in tragedy, the mother typically grieves more intensely and for a longer time. But a father can also grieve deeply, although he may hide his emotions because he feels socially constrained or wants to be 'strong' for his partner.

As you become acquainted with your grief, try to be patient with yourself and understand that mourning a pregnancy loss takes time. Expressing your feelings about your loss is an important part of grief. You may be helped by having someone to talk or cry with, whether it be your partner, another family member, a friend, a member of the clergy, a psychotherapist, or other bereaved parents in a support group. Consider asking your obstetrician to contact other parents who have suffered a similar loss to see if they would be willing to talk with you. If you wish, try keeping a journal, tape-record your thoughts and feelings, or write a letter or poem to your baby. You may also want to read comforting books and poems, or the sort of newsletter produced by support groups such as BLISS, SANDS or SATEA. Expressing your sorrow does not lessen your loss, but it can help you mourn and allow your grief to resolve gradually.

There are several other practical things you can do to help you survive this sad time. Respect your own inclinations about whether to put away baby things yourself or have others do this for you. If you feel a religious ceremony would be meaningful, consider planning and participating in a ceremony to mark your loss, even if it is only a simple one at home for your immediate family. Try to pamper yourself for a while, too. Ask for help with household chores or with your other children, and avoid social situations with expectant couples or infants until you are ready to handle them.

Grief is physically depleting, so try to eat regular, balanced meals and organize some form of exercise every day. Get lots of rest, even if you have trouble sleeping. As tempting as alcohol may be, you should avoid drinking, since it can impede the grieving process and, as a depressant, will only make you feel worse. If your sadness is not improving, or if you are feeling worse two to three months after your loss, consider seeing a psychotherapist for bereavement counselling. If necessary, she can refer you to a doctor for medication to relieve depression or help you sleep.

Although you may long for a change in your life immediately after your loss, you should keep in mind that grief impairs judgment. It is preferable to avoid making major decisions, such as a job change or move, until both you and your partner feel more emotionally settled, usually about a year after your loss. With time, as you mourn, you should begin to feel better and to look forward to your future with hope.

Whatever stage of grief you are in right now, you will probably go through various aspects of grief in the months ahead. Phases of grief can pass and then return again. Although you will grieve in your own unique way and your grief will have its own life, rhythm, and eventual resolution, you may find it helpful to learn about the typical phases of grief and the feelings each may bring.

Shock and Denial

When you lose your pregnancy, you may cry uncontrollably at first and then experience emotional shock and denial, feeling numb and detached, unable to believe the pregnancy has really ended. Emotional shock is probably a self-protective response that allows you to mobilize internal strength to cope with your tragedy. It may last several hours or days, or it may come and go over a few weeks.

During emotional shock, you may feel you are in the midst of a bad dream from which you hope to awaken to find a healthy pregnancy or a live baby. Although you probably remember exactly how you learned about your loss, you may not recall other conversations or events that took place while you were in this initial state of shock.

Adam experienced this phase of grief as soon as his wife's doctor diagnosed their baby's severe genetic defect two weeks before her due date:

> He told us that our baby was anencephalic, that she didn't have a fully formed skull or brain and would not survive long after birth. Lisa let out a horrible shriek and broke into tears, crying hysterically. She fell into my arms, and I started crying with her. Everything we had hoped for in the nine months was taken away in that split second.
>
> While we made the arrangements to have a funeral and bury the baby, my attitude was one of total shock. And that time period between our daughter's death and when she was buried is a complete loss and blank period for us both.

If you suffered a loss early in your pregnancy, you can feel equally stunned, even if only a few days or weeks have elapsed since you learned about the conception. The baby you had just begun to anticipate is suddenly no longer there. Being jolted from the elation of the initial news to the sorrow of the loss can be staggering at a time when you already feel vulnerable from a new pregnancy.

Ellen was in the ninth week of her first pregnancy when she awoke in the middle of the night, bleeding profusely. As her husband searched the early-morning streets for a taxi to take her to the hospital, she waited alone in their flat.

> At that point I was just astounded by what was happening. Even the ride to the hospital, with the taxi driver rushing through red lights, seemed surreal. It wasn't until the next morning, after the miscarriage

was over, that I fully realized we were not going to be parents.

A mother who experiences a midterm or late pregnancy loss can develop disturbing symptoms during this initial stage of emotional shock. She may imagine she hears the hungry wails of her deceased baby, a phenomenon called 'phantom crying,' or she may feel a kicking sensation in her womb after delivery. The bereaved mother knows these sensations are impossible, and she may wonder if she is losing her mind, but they are normal reactions to a traumatic loss and should subside with time.

Dr Kenneth Kellner, an obstetrician who has researched the needs of bereaved parents, found that mothers who heard phantom crying or imagined the baby kicking usually stopped having these sensations when they were allowed to see, hold, and say goodbye to their babies. Some care-givers have also noted that if a mother no longer has these options, she usually stops hearing phantom crying when she can at least see her baby's photograph.

You may find that episodes of numbness and denial come and go, but they eventually disappear, especially if you are given the chance to grieve your loss openly.

Anticipatory Grief

If you learn that your baby has died before the actual miscarriage or delivery, you may experience a phase of sorrow called anticipatory grief, in which you begin to mourn while the baby is still in the womb. Yet, even as you start to mourn, you may be unable to believe fully that the pregnancy has ended until it is physically over. One woman, whose baby stopped growing twelve weeks into the pregnancy, had a dilatation and curettage, or D&C, to remove the ended pregnancy. 'I was in mourning from the moment I knew the baby had died,' she explained. 'But it really hit me after the D&C. Then it was final.'

If your baby was born gravely ill or dying, you probably began to grieve when you learned about your baby's condition. If you had antenatal testing that diagnosed a severe abnormality in your unborn baby, you probably began to mourn as you awaited the abortion. Your feelings of anger, anxiety, and depression probably intensified as the delivery, or the death, approached.

With the pregnancy finally over and your remnants of hope or disbelief gone, you may feel a confusing mixture of sadness at the loss and relief that your agonizing uncertainty has ended. As the reality of your loss sinks in, you can begin to mourn fully.

Acute Grief

As shock and denial recede, the enormity of your tragedy may hit you full force, plunging you into acute grief. The emotional and physical upheaval you experience when your loss is new can be all consuming and may last from several days to several weeks. It can be frightening to feel such emotional pain and to be so out of control. Crying fits and nightmares are common during acute grief, as are physical complaints such as insomnia, extreme fatigue, digestive problems, tightness in the throat, and shortness of breath.

While you are still very raw from your loss, you may find you cannot function well. You may be unable to concentrate on even simple tasks and may feel little energy for your usual activities, including work, care of your other children, maintaining your personal appearance, or socializing.

After Sarah's first baby was stillborn, all she could manage to do was watch TV and lie in bed:

> I wasn't able to do anything else. We cut ourselves off from others, folded into ourselves. Then I wouldn't eat, wouldn't get dressed, couldn't function. I couldn't even get out of bed to make myself breakfast! This lasted three or four weeks.

You may find that all you think about is your pregnancy loss as you review in your mind, over and over, all the details of the tragedy. You may also experience a terrible sense of failure. As one woman who had two consecutive miscarriages put it, 'Everyone can have babies, and I can't. I feel it is a terrible defect in me.'

The overwhelming emotions of acute grief can be frightening. At times you may feel so dysfunctional, so upset and out of control, you may begin to wonder if you are losing your mind. But most likely you are experiencing a normal, albeit distressing aspect of acute grief.

Amy had an early miscarriage, which she never mourned, followed quickly by a subsequent pregnancy, which ended in another early loss. Her grief over both losses hit her at once, together with her fears that she would never have a baby, and she began to fear for her sanity:

> There were a few times after the second loss when I felt I was going crazy. I would sit on my bed and stare for hours and cry uncontrollably. It was scary.

During acute grief, some parents have transient thoughts of wanting to die, as a desperate expression of their wish to rejoin their baby. Although these thoughts are frightening, they are not unusual. However, it is very important for bereaved parents to share these feelings with a supportive family member or friend. If troubling thoughts and feelings continue, it is crucial to seek psychotherapy for support during this stressful time.

You may feel anxious and vulnerable after your tragedy, fearing that another loved one will come to harm. You may become very aware of the fragility of life and overly protective of yourself and your family. You may even have to struggle to let your family engage in normal activities, which suddenly seem dangerous.

Christine became terribly anxious for the safety of her family after she suffered a stillbirth:

> At first I was afraid whenever someone left the house that they would die, both children and husband. I felt overprotective. It was a real struggle to let my son even ride his bike to school.

Anxiety and overprotectiveness are understandable responses to a pregnancy loss and should ease with time as your mourning process continues.

Within two or three months of your loss, you may find your physical and emotional turmoil begin to subside. You no longer constantly picture the details of your tragedy, as you did in the early weeks after your loss. You might be able to resume work and household responsibilities, perhaps you cry less often, and your eating and sleeping patterns become more regular. However, it may seem that you are 'going through the motions' rather than being fully involved with your activities. Preoccupation with the loss and feelings of depression can continue to dominate your life.

Unfortunately, you may find that many people expect you to be over your grief within a couple of months. They may interpret your return to work or to other activities as a sign that you are feeling fine. You might encounter remarks such as, 'Put the loss behind you, and get on with your life,' or 'It's been three months now. Why are you still depressed?'

Though feelings of grief are usually less constant and debilitating several weeks after a loss, mourning can continue for several months and may last a year or more. The lack of understanding from others may add to the upset and isolation you already feel, a topic explored more fully in Chapter 11, 'The Response of Your Family and Friends.'

Anger, Guilt, and Blame

At some point following your loss, your sadness may be tinged with feelings of anger and guilt or a wish to blame someone. These feelings usually have nothing to do with any real fault; they are an understandable attempt to make sense out of a senseless tragedy. No matter what caused the loss, you may condemn yourself, your partner, your doctor, or even God.

Hilary conceived twins in her first pregnancy and felt fine until she noticed slight bleeding in her sixth month. When she learned at the hospital that her cervix had opened and the delivery could not be stopped, she became furious with the doctor who told her the babies could not be saved:

> The obstetrician said, 'There is nothing we can do. One baby is in the birth canal.' I hated this man. I lashed out at him every time he came in. I thought, 'Maybe he's wrong.' I needed someone to be angry at.

You may also feel angry at how terribly unfair your loss is. You may read about neglected children, or unfit parents, and feel the injustice of not having the child you want so badly while others have children they don't seem to want or care for. As one bereaved father admitted:

> I had a lot of hostility. I felt deprived of my baby and of fatherhood. Looking at other people who had what I didn't have made me wonder, 'Why can this idiot have a family and children and I can't?' This was a question I asked myself a lot.

At the same time, you may worry that you are in some way to blame for your loss and may mentally search for things you might have done to cause it. You may wonder, for example, if your loss is a punishment for not planning your pregnancy or for considering an abortion. Even if you always intended to keep the pregnancy, you may worry that ambivalence about it, or your preference for a child of one sex or the other, caused the loss. Wishes and ambivalence have never caused a pregnancy loss, but these worries can torment you.

Stuart, whose wife experienced an early loss in their first – and unplanned – pregnancy, wondered if their miscarriage was a punishment for their doubts:

> We were young, we hadn't been married very long, and we were worried that our ambivalence toward the pregnancy might have

caused the loss, that we hadn't wanted the baby enough.

In struggling to comprehend your loss, you may fault yourself for taking a trip or having sexual relations immediately before your pregnancy ended, neither of which is likely to cause harm. Your feelings of self-blame may be so strong that you become convinced you should be punished in some way.

Sarah intentionally refused medication through the painful delivery of her stillborn son because she felt she deserved to suffer after his death was confirmed. Only later did her husband, Roger, learn her reasons:

> The labour took a long time, even with Syntocinon to speed it up and Sarah was in a lot of pain. The doctor said, 'Don't be a hero, take something for the pain,' but she refused. Later she told me she felt she had to punish herself. If I had known that, I would have demanded she take some medication. It seemed so unfair for her to be blaming herself like that.

It is natural to wonder if you could have somehow protected your pregnancy. Unfounded guilt can intensify, especially if your need to grieve and talk about your loss goes unacknowledged. While feelings of guilt are common, it is highly unlikely that anything you did or neglected to do actually caused your pregnancy loss. And it is crucial for you to raise any questions or fears with your doctor, because the medical facts are often reassuring.

Ellen was sure she had caused her first miscarriage, a fear that persisted until she directly questioned her obstetrician:

> I hoovered the house the day before I started having cramping pains and couldn't erase the fear that doing the heavy cleaning that day had caused the miscarriage. I was relieved when the doctor confirmed that the baby had probably died a couple of weeks earlier.

A mother who experiences a loss from a medical condition she didn't know about, such as cervical incompetence or an undiagnosed hormonal imbalance, may feel guilty that her body did not sustain the pregnancy. It is important for her to try not to be too hard on herself for something neither she, nor her doctor, knew to prevent. Finding out what precautions to take during any subsequent pregnancy can help her guilt feelings subside.

Guilt can be a severe problem for parents who engaged in activities or who were exposed to substances that can actually harm a pregnancy. A man may feel responsible if he discovers his exposure to toxic substances at work could have caused his wife's miscarriages. Similarly, a woman who smoked heavily during her pregnancy, and lost the baby due to prematurity, may worry that her smoking was a contributing factor.

If you feel responsible for a loss because your pregnancy was exposed to harmful substances, your guilt can paralyse you emotionally and prevent you from grieving. Try to make any necessary changes that will allow you to take realistic precautions for your next pregnancy. It is important to realize you don't have to handle this difficult situation by yourself. Psychotherapy can enable you to make changes and to forgive yourself for dangers you were unaware of before the loss, or for behaviours that were out of your control.

Guilt can also be a source of great distress if you underwent antenatal testing and chose to abort an abnormal pregnancy. No matter how strongly you feel that you made the right choice, being forced to choose places an additional burden on you. This is a particularly agonizing experience, which is explored more fully in Chapter 8, 'Antenatal Diagnosis and Abortion: The Burden of Choice.'

Searching and Yearning for Your Baby

You might find yourself searching and yearning for your baby weeks or months after the loss. You may constantly imagine what you would now be doing with the baby and become uncomfortably aware of every infant you encounter who was born near your own due date. Longing for your child can be a way of wishing to undo the finality of the loss. This happened to Hilary, whose premature twins died at birth:

> For a long time I would fantasize about the babies, putting them into situations. I would go into a supermarket and think, 'I couldn't fit a double buggy in here.' When driving I would think the twins should be in the back seat.
>
> Once on a business trip I told a fellow passenger I had twins. I'm really embarrassed about this. I engaged in this fantasy and pretended they had lived. It was so nice. The man was kind and I knew I would never see him again.

Yearning for your baby can also take the form of longing to become pregnant again quickly, which is a natural response to the void created by a loss. But when either you or your partner desperately wants to conceive again, you may be wishing that the loss could be undone rather than feeling ready for another pregnancy. One woman conveyed her urgent desire for a baby after two miscarriages when she told her husband, 'I have waited for such a long time to have kids. I have to have one! Get me one!'

While the wish to replace the baby is understandable, it is important for you to mourn your loss before embarking on a new pregnancy. If you conceive straight after a loss, you may be unable to grieve, because mourning your loss and bonding with a new pregnancy are demanding and opposite emotional tasks, difficult to do at the same time. If you give yourself time to grieve your loss, you will eventually realize that another pregnancy will not replace the baby who died, enabling you to welcome the baby who follows into your family as a new and unique individual. You may read more about pregnancy following a loss in Chapter 16, 'Becoming Pregnant Again.'

Jealousy

At the beginning it seemed that every time I turned on the TV someone was having a baby – on the news, on shows. The world was full of pregnant women. Everything reminded me of the baby.

MAGGIE

After your loss, it may seem as if babies and pregnant women are everywhere, from TV advertisements to expectant couples on the street, triggering an immediate, gut response of both jealousy and hurt. Even if you had never paid attention to children before, you may find you have become painfully aware of babies everywhere you go. Derek, who lost premature twins, remarked, 'Everywhere I went I saw twins, which never happened before.'

You may be especially troubled by your envy because it does not fit your self-image and can alienate you from friends or relatives you care about. You may criticize yourself for feeling angry with a pregnant sister-in-law or for avoiding friends with new babies.

It is important for you to realize that most bereaved parents experience these feelings and reactions. Jealousy of expectant parents after a loss is no reflection on your character, but rather an understandable and temporary aspect of grief.

You cannot avoid seeing babies and pregnant couples on the street sometimes. But you can take care of yourself by explaining to friends or relatives who are either pregnant or new parents that you cannot see them for a while because of your loss. If they care about you, they will respect your wishes, and you can let them know when you feel ready to socialize again.

Acceptance of the Loss and Anniversary Reactions

A time will eventually come when you begin to feel real relief and are no longer constantly and painfully reminded of your loss. In the course of remembering and talking about your tragedy, you will gradually come to terms with it, a process that can take months, a year, or even longer. 'Time helped,' recalled Derek. 'It took at least one year before we could talk about the loss without getting all emotional.'

Once time has passed, you may start to feel as if a weight has been lifted from you. You find your appetite and sleep patterns are returning to normal. You may take renewed pleasure in family, work, and recreation and once again enjoy socializing. You can expect to continue to think about your loss, but daily activities and plans for your future will become important as well. The painful emotions of mourning will re-emerge from time to time, but the feelings may be short-lived and less intense.

If you suffered a late pregnancy loss, or the death of a newborn, you may experience guilt as you start to feel better, as if grief were loyalty to your baby and relief tantamount to abandonment or betrayal of your child. It is important to realize that you can let go of your pain and still be faithful to memories of your baby and to the special place that baby has in your heart.

You may find that your mourning feels more resolved only when you become a parent, through childbirth or adoption. While the new baby cannot replace the one you lost, the demands and pleasures of having an infant, and your affirmation as a parent, may help you continue the healing process that began with active mourning. But memories of the pregnancy loss remain. Joel found this to be true when his healthy son was born:

> Everything has changed for me since Sam was born. The pain of losing our daughter diminished more. However, there are times when I see Sam and think of our daughter. It is bittersweet.

Couples who do not have the solace of becoming parents may need to find other ways to resolve their feelings of loss. They face special emotional challenges that are discussed in Chapter 15, 'Pregnancy Loss and Infertility: A Twofold Loss.'

Anniversaries of the due date, birth, or death often bring on a brief resurgence of grief, known as an 'anniversary reaction.' Other reminders of the baby, including another pregnancy and birth, can have the same effect. 'I still cry around her birthday,' explained Lisa three years after her infant daughter died from congenital defects. 'I cried for her when my son was born, and at Christmas. Sometimes I cry when I see baby things in shops, little dresses for little girls. Things like that.'

As an anniversary approaches, you may become depressed, tearful, and preoccupied by your loss, much as you felt immediately after the tragedy. An anniversary reaction can be disconcerting, especially if you are unprepared for it. 'I was doing much better,' said one woman. 'Now I am irritable and tearful again.' Another mother noted, 'The anniversary of the stillbirth is coming up and it's always on my mind.'

If you suffered an early loss, you may experience two anniversary reactions in a year, one at the due date and the other a year after the loss. Karen remembered all five due dates from each of her first-trimester losses. 'I think of the babies as each due date comes and goes,' she admitted. 'I think of how old those babies would be now and how close or far apart they would be in relationship to my two children.' Usually when the anniversary has passed, the upset also subsides and you again feel better.

If You Have Difficulty Mourning

It is natural, although painful, to grieve after a pregnancy loss, but it is not altogether automatic. Mourning can either be supported or inhibited by your own tendencies to acknowledge or suppress feelings. Your ability to grieve can also be greatly affected by the reactions of others. If you do not mourn effectively, your grief may go underground and interfere with your mood, relationships, or functioning for a long time after your loss.

If you fail to grieve, the symptoms of mourning can become chronic. Feelings of depression and worthlessness as well as nightmares or overactivity can persist for many months without improvement. If you become chronically bereaved, you may experience persistent crying spells, irritability, or anxiety, and you may sleep and eat too little or too much. Chronic bereavement can lead to a breakdown in your sexual and marital relationships, and it can leave you functioning poorly at work or unable to enjoy recreation. You may even develop stress-related medical problems.

Although any grieving parent may experience these symptoms, if you become chronically bereaved you do not recover from your sorrow as well as you might, primarily because you do not have outlets to express your grief.

You may even be unaware that your troubling symptoms are related to your pregnancy loss, because you have denied and repressed your thoughts and feelings.

Many factors can prevent you from grieving as you need to. If you do not realize your upset is a natural response to the loss, or if your family, friends, and health care providers are intolerant of your grief, you may have difficulty mourning.

Laura delivered a very premature baby in the hospital, but no staff were in the room with her at the time. After the birth, a nurse arrived and removed the infant without speaking to Laurel or showing her the baby. The nursing staff continued to avoid her until her discharge.

In retrospect, Laura realized it took her a long time to begin to grieve because of the lack of support in the hospital. 'I went home feeling like a freak because no one wanted to talk to me,' she explained. 'The hospital tried to make it all go away. I kept feeling that was what I had to do: make it all go away.'

You can also develop a chronic grief response if you had a midterm or late pregnancy loss but did not see your baby or say goodbye. Ruth had suffered an early miscarriage and then a pregnancy loss at five months. When her second loss occurred, she did not look at her baby, and she plunged into a busy work routine straight afterwards, both of which prevented her from mourning:

> After losing the baby, I thought I was doing okay and threw myself back into my old routine. But then I started having inappropriate behaviour at strange times. I would start crying suddenly or show lots of anger and not know where the sadness and anger were coming from. Then I realized things weren't okay, and I tracked down the hospital social worker, who told me about SANDS. I finally allowed myself to grieve.

With the help of the group, Ruth's suppressed feelings surfaced. She needed to grieve her losses and to grieve not having seen or held her baby. She also had to deal with worries about having a successful pregnancy in the future. As she and her husband talked out their feelings and fears in the group and at home, Ruth's crying spells and angry outbursts subsided and eventually stopped.

Another circumstance that can cause chronic grief occurs when the pregnancy loss rekindles sadness over an earlier emotional trauma, such as the previous death of a loved one. Caroline was plunged into a severe depression when she lost a premature baby boy and became terrified that her healthy older son would also die. Her depression improved when she sought psychotherapy and worked through old fears stemming from a childhood tragedy, when her younger brother had died in a drowning accident. 'The loss of my baby son brought back my childhood nightmare,' she recalled, 'that little boys die.'

Grief can also become blocked and chronic when there is a multiple gestation, such as twins, and one baby dies while the other survives. If this happened to you, your love and wish to care for the surviving baby, and the infant's demands on you, make it especially difficult to mourn the twin who died. Kristen Swanson-Kauffman, a nurse, explains how confusing and ambivalent new parenthood can be in this situation:

> Congratulations and condolences and birth and death announce-ments, are all a part of the first few postpartum weeks. While trying to bond to the surviving twin, parents are also experiencing the need to grieve the dead twin.

If you are the parent of a surviving twin, you may be confused and angered by people who tell you that you should be happy that one baby lived. You may also find you cannot grieve effectively because you are caring for the surviving infant. 'I feel I'm in mourning all the time,' explained Nora after one of her twins was stillborn. 'But I can't really let myself mourn because I have my son to tend to.'

Special grieving problems continue for you as your baby grows. Every joy for the surviving twin, every milestone and holiday is a happy occasion with a shadow cast over it because of the absent twin.

If you lost a twin, you need and deserve support for the constant challenges and difficulties you face. Psychotherapy and bereavement support groups can help. There is also a bereavement support group attached to the Twin and Multiple Births Association (TAMBA).

If you are unable to mourn on your own, you can get help to complete the grieving process. You need an environment in which you can safely express your grief and fears, whether by opening communication with your partner, by joining a bereavement support group, by engaging in psychotherapy, or by a combination of these outlets. You may need to backtrack and talk about earlier sorrows that have resurfaced as a result of your pregnancy loss. With time and with adequate understanding and support, you can be helped to tolerate your grief and allow it to resolve.

Pregnancy Loss Changes You

You may discover that your pregnancy loss leaves a permanent mark on you. In addition to the sad consequences, you may notice other changes that are positive and meaningful, such as a greater sensitivity to others who experience a loss, or a deeper appreciation for loved ones. You may re-evaluate your personal goals and make a career change, or you might make new commitments to community responsibilities you feel are worthwhile.

Susannah found that she experienced many changes after her miscarriages and the subsequent birth of her son:

> A loss changes you forever, it touches you forever, and you never forget it. It makes you appreciate your children more. Having a child is so much more important than other things in life.
>
> Even going back to school to get my degree was a gift from my 'other children' and grew out of my losses. People who haven't experienced losses just never really understand this. It has been a real character – well, addition, for lack of another word. I'm more willing to overlook a lot of things I wouldn't have before. I am more forgiving of people.

As time passes and as the more active stages of mourning come to a close, you will probably feel renewed energy and interest in yourself, your family, and your daily life. But the loss remains a permanent part of your life and history and is never forgotten.

What Can Help You Grieve

Grief is a natural and necessary response to your pregnancy loss and is a physically and emotionally exhausting process. It is very important that you give yourself permission to grieve and that you have adequate support during this difficult time. The grieving process takes longer than most people expect, often six months to one year or more before the pain and preoccupation with the loss subside.

Here are some suggestions to help you manage the painful, confusing, and sometimes overwhelming emotions of the mourning process:

- Grief can be expressed by talking, remembering, or crying over your loss and the baby. Try to find understanding listeners – a loved one, a friend, a member of the clergy, a psychotherapist, or a support group. Consider asking your obstetrician to put you in touch with other parents who have had a similar loss. You might want to write down or tape record your thoughts and feelings, or compose a letter or poem to your baby.

- It is important to take care of your health, as grief is physically depleting. Try to eat regular, balanced meals, avoid alcohol, maintain your usual rest patterns even if you have trouble sleeping, and get some exercise daily if you are able.

- When possible, postpone any major decisions, such as a job change or move, for about one year after a loss. The emotional turmoil of grief may make a change in your circumstances seem appealing, but grief impairs judgment, and it is preferable to avoid significant changes until you feel better.

- Consider reading comforting literature such as books on pregnancy loss, or poetry that make you feel understood. For parents who have lost a twin, consider contacting the bereavement support group of TAMBA, the Twins and Multiple Birth Association. For other suggested reading, see Appendix D.

- With time, your mood should improve. Signs that you are healing emotionally include returning to your usual appetite and sleep patterns, having increased energy for your daily routine, being able to feel happy without feeling guilty, taking pleasure in your family relationships and in social contacts, and, when alone, regaining an ability to think about things other than the loss.

- You may want to consider bereavement counselling if you need more support than you can find informally, if your depression is worsening or not improving two to three months after a loss, or if you are not satisfied with your emotional progress at any point after your loss. It is especially important to locate a psychotherapist who understands this type of loss and who can give you the extra support you deserve during your bereavement.

CHAPTER 2
. . . .

THE MOTHER'S EXPERIENCE

When your pregnancy ends in loss, both you and the baby's father suffer. However, your experience of the loss, as well as your emotional expression, are probably quite different from his. You physically carried this baby and experienced the major hormonal changes that follow a loss. Moreover, your deep-seated childhood expectations of one day becoming a mother may have nurtured your dreams of parenthood for years. You have to deal with the loss of those childhood dreams, at least for now, as well as the emotional and physical impact of losing your expected baby. Because of your unique relation to the pregnancy, you will probably grieve your loss more openly and for a longer time than the baby's father.

Factors That Affect Your Grief

Physical, hormonal, and emotional factors all contribute to the deep sense of sorrow and the relatively lengthy grieving period you may experience following your pregnancy loss. You physically carried and nurtured your baby from the moment of conception and probably bonded to the pregnancy in both conscious and unconscious ways. You may not have realized that your body responded to your conception immediately with major hormonal shifts, so you were probably unprepared for the sudden physical changes triggered by your loss, even an early miscarriage. Your morning sickness suddenly disappeared, your breasts were no longer tender, and that mysterious and wonderful glow people may have mentioned to you had gone from your face.

The further along you were in your pregnancy, the more complicated your body's response to your loss. These changes may continue for weeks afterward and may be associated with such real events as your milk – a devastating reminder of the absent baby – or the onset of your first menstrual period following your loss.

These same abrupt hormonal shifts can often provoke normal postnatal 'blues' following the delivery of a healthy baby. When your loss occurred, your body went through the same sudden reduction in hormones, but there was neither a baby to rejoice in nor happy relatives and friends to offer congratulations, help, or support. Instead, your body and heart were preparing to mother, and there was no baby to be mothered. As Lisa recalled, following the birth of her full-term baby who lived only a few hours, 'I remember standing in the shower when my milk came in and I just stood there crying. The baby had died, but my body didn't know it.'

Your desire to nurture and parent your baby, the bond that was built hour by hour as you felt your growing baby's presence, continues after your loss as a bond of grief. You may feel you have lost not only your baby but also part of yourself, as if a vital portion of your own body were missing. Your sense of emptiness can be especially overwhelming if you have no other children, because then you have lost the dream of motherhood, at least for a time, as well as this baby.

When you suffer this double loss, of baby and motherhood, a sense of failure can spill over into other areas of your life and affect your entire self-concept. Natalie had two early miscarriages, and then a loss at nineteen weeks, which profoundly undermined her feelings of self-worth:

> I feel constantly preoccupied by the losses. I have this yearning for motherhood. I have this feeling of deprivation, inadequacy, sadness. I need constant reminders that this doesn't declare me incompetent as a person because I am not a mother. The desire, the wanting to have a baby and not being able to have one is excruciating.

If your loss is made worse by a sense of failure, try to focus on the ways you took care of your unborn baby even if you experienced normal ambivalence during the pregnancy. Perhaps you gave up smoking or alcohol when you decided to conceive, or as soon as you learned you were pregnant. You may have improved your diet or sought the best obstetric care possible. If you endured a medical crisis during your pregnancy, your sacrifices of time and effort to maintain the pregnancy may have been enormous. Even though you couldn't prevent your loss, all of the consideration and commitment you gave your pregnancy are proof that you were a good and loving mother to your unborn child.

You can also help keep negative feelings about yourself from overwhelming you if you try to concentrate on your strengths and abilities following your loss. Even small accomplishments can bolster your self-confidence without denying your need to grieve and may allow feelings of loss, not failure, to come forward and resolve themselves. Re-read a work report you are proud of, or have lunch with a friend. Try to draw on your talents, even though doing so may seem frivolous at first, and take the time to reach out to people you care about and whom you know care about you.

After her fourth miscarriage, one mother recalled writing a series of letters to friends she had not been in touch with for several months:

> I pride myself on my letter writing and found that sending the letters had a very positive effect on my mood. I didn't even mention my most recent loss in all the letters. I wasn't looking for sympathy. I was looking more for a small feeling of fulfilment that involved people I loved.

Taking the time to pamper yourself can also help you maintain a positive attitude toward yourself amid the sorrow of your loss. If you usually wear makeup and enjoy dressing nicely, try to continue taking care of your appearance. Treat yourself to a facial or a massage. Think about simple activities that have given you satisfaction in the past, such as going to see a film, cooking, or exercising, and do your best to make time for them, even if you are having trouble concentrating. If you continue to give yourself positive outlets and support, any negative feelings about yourself will be less likely to grow out of proportion.

Feeling You Failed the Baby's Father

Both you and the baby's father may have planned to share the responsibility for the care and upbringing of your children. The significant changes in societal expectations about child-rearing and sexual role models that came about in the 1960s and 1970s may have had a profound effect on your decision to adjust each of your careers jointly to make room for a baby in your lives.

Yet like many women, you may have found pregnancy conferred on you a special status because of your unique physical role. No matter how equally you and your partner shared decisions about having and raising a child, you may have felt very special as you carried, nurtured, and felt love for your child, experiencing at the same time a deepening bond between you and the baby's father.

When you lost your pregnancy, you may have lost this special relationship to your partner. Julia and Ian had one little boy and were expecting their second child when Julia's uterus ruptured almost at term, causing the baby's death. Although her life had been endangered by her medical condition, she still felt guilty because she thought she had deprived her husband of a second child. 'I feel terrible,' she explained. 'He's a wonderful father. He should have had a second son, and I feel it's my fault that he doesn't have one.' Sometimes a childless woman even contemplates divorce so her husband could remarry and have children more easily, regardless of the husband's devotion to her and commitment to the marriage.

This twofold experience of 'failure' as mother and wife can intensify your grief and complicate your emotional recovery from the loss. It is important to keep communication open so that you and your partner talk about these concerns and deal with them as you need to, rather than keeping them private and letting them fester.

The Ways Women Grieve

As a woman you may feel a compelling need to talk or cry about your pregnancy loss with compassionate listeners. Talking can help you express your grief, leaving you deeply appreciative of others who listen to you and understand you.

But coping with a pregnancy loss may also leave you feeling selfish for concentrating so intensely on your own preoccupations. Our society encourages women to care for the needs and feelings of others, often before their own, so it may be difficult for you to make time for your sorrow. Although it may seem self-centred to want to focus on your own distress after the loss, this is an important step in coming to terms with your grief.

Women who grieve openly may notice that their emotional style is different from their partner's more reserved response. This tendency is reinforced by our culture, which expects women to be emotional while men are not supposed to show feelings. Maggie observed that she and her husband had very different reactions to their premature baby's delivery and death:

> We both felt very sad about the loss, but as a woman, I was more emotional and I would cry and Bert would be comforting. I also did more of the talking and initiated most of the conversations about my feelings.

Regardless of your partner's way of expressing his sorrow, if you feel the need to talk about your loss, by all means seek out an understanding family member, close friend, or member of the clergy who will listen sympathetically, because talking can help your emotional recovery. If you don't know anyone you can comfortably talk to, you may find meeting with a sensitive psychotherapist extremely helpful. Attending a bereaved parents' support group, if one exists in your area, can be especially beneficial, as it provides the companionship of others who know what your loss is like.

Your Return to the Community

Returning to work or your usual activities in the community can be difficult after a pregnancy loss. With an early loss, if you had not yet told colleagues or friends you were expecting, you may feel awkward telling them you miscarried. Nevertheless, you will probably feel better if you tell some friends about your loss so you can get support during the difficult weeks of adjustment that follow. If you are back at work, it may be a good idea to let a few sympathetic colleagues know what you have been through so they can make allowances for your being moody or distracted.

One mother, who was physically well enough to return to work a few days after her miscarriage, found the emotional pressure of feeling alone with her misfortune almost unbearable. 'I'd be sitting at my desk and want to stand up and scream, "I had a baby and was pregnant and now it's gone!"' she recalled. 'I wish I had told people earlier along. I needed that extra support.'

If your pregnancy was showing, your return to work or other activities will probably involve frequent reminders of your loss. Colleagues and neighbours will probably ask about your baby and you will have to tell the sad news, sometimes when you have no desire to discuss it. Some people will be genuinely concerned and others merely curious.

Hilary lost premature twins and was so upset by questions when she returned to work that she stopped trying to give polite answers:

> I went back to work six months after our loss. I work for a large firm, so most of my colleagues only knew I had been out on maternity leave and said, 'Oh, you're back. What did you have?' Sometimes I was mean and just bluntly said, 'They died.'

Once back in your usual routine, you will inevitably encounter pregnant women, mothers, and babies, and each confrontation can reawaken feelings of hurt and failure. Sylvia, whose full-term baby died shortly after birth, worked for a travel agency that maintained several offices in her area. She arranged to switch locations when she returned to work, so her colleagues wouldn't know about her pregnancy or her loss and she could tell only those she wanted to. But this did not protect her as much as she had hoped:

> They changed my location, but they put me in an office where many young mothers and babies came in. One mother came up to my desk with her new baby and asked if I wanted to hold it. I said 'No,' and ran crying to the bathroom. I spent a lot of time crying in that bathroom over the next six months.

Once you accept that your emotional response to these awkward situations is to be expected, you can begin to forgive yourself and allow your grief to surface. For a fuller discussion of how to handle these predicaments, please read Chapter 11, 'The Response of Your Family and Friends.'

What Can Help Bereaved Mothers

Grief over your pregnancy loss may include sorrow for your baby and your lost chance to mother this child, as well as grief for an aspect of your womanhood. You should not have to go through this misfortune alone. You need and deserve opportunities to talk over your thoughts and feelings about the pregnancy, your tragedy, and what these meant to you. You need others to listen who appreciate the magnitude of your loss, because sharing your experience with sympathetic listeners can validate your feelings. When you talk about your loss you make a statement, for you and for those you speak with, that the pregnancy was important and real.

Here are some additional suggestions to help you cope with your particular sorrow:

- You may experience an intense and fairly prolonged grief reaction because you physically carried the baby you lost and your expectations of becoming a mother are so deeply engrained. Give yourself the time and outlets you need to mourn properly.
- If you find yourself succumbing to a sense of failure as a woman following your loss, try to concentrate on your areas of competence as

you continue to grieve, allowing the feelings of loss, not failure, to come forward and resolve.

- If you feel reluctant to place your sorrow before the feelings and demands of others, try to remember that expressing your grief is an important part of coming to terms with your loss and that you need and deserve to take good care of yourself during your bereavement.
- Your partner may not appear depressed because he is busy keeping the home going and relieved that you are in good health. Do not assume, however, that this means he lacks feelings about the pregnancy loss. It may simply be hard for him to express his sorrow.
- Try to accept the conflicting emotions you may experience when you return to work and your regular routine. Acknowledge the difficult feelings aroused by seeing pregnant women and mothers with young children. These are understandable reactions that should diminish with time.

CHAPTER 3

·············

THE FATHER'S EXPERIENCE

As a husband and father, it has probably been extremely difficult for you to feel so helpless in the face of your family's loss. You may see yourself as a provider who must focus his energies on constructive action, such as returning to a busy work schedule or caring for other children at home. Although these activities are an important help to your family during the crisis, they may divert you from your anger and sadness, feelings that can seem unacceptable to men. By concentrating on your partner's recovery and by feeling relief as she physically regains her strength, you may also be deflecting your thoughts away from your own grief.

On the other hand, if you are a father who tends to express his feelings openly by crying and talking to family and friends, you may have encountered other people's discomfort when you displayed your emotions. At a time when you needed understanding and support, this unspoken criticism may have felt like an added injury.

You may also be troubled by having to take care of so many practical details following the loss, leaving you guilt-ridden for worrying about mundane problems when faced with such a monumental sorrow. Watching your partner suffer may only increase your sadness and frustration. 'It was so hard for me to deal with my wife's milk coming in,' remembered Simon, whose first child was stillborn. 'It made me feel so completely helpless.'

Bonding With Your Baby

As a bereaved father, your experience of the pregnancy and the loss can be quite different from the mother's. If you had a first-trimester loss, hearing the heartbeat and seeing an early scan could have brought home the reality of the pregnancy, but you may have had no other direct experience of the baby. Your feelings of loss may have related more to the disruption of your plans for a family and to your partner's distress, and less to feelings about the baby. With either a miscarriage or a late loss you may be like some fathers who feel the full impact of the pregnancy only as the birth – and death – occur.

If you suffered a stillbirth or newborn death, you likely felt shock and disbelief at first, and then the anguish of your loss. You probably had to pull yourself together quickly to make needed arrangements with the hospital or mortuary and to plan for your wife's sad homecoming. Whether your loss was early or full-term, your attachment to the baby may not be the same as your partner's, because hers was physical as well as emotional. As one bereaved husband explained to his wife after their full-term baby died:

> You carried her and knew her the best for nine months. I didn't feel every kick and turn. It's not that I didn't love her or have hopes for her. But I didn't live with her the way you did.

While the mother's bond with the baby is usually stronger than the father's, there are important exceptions. Some men develop substantial physical and emotional attachments to their infants by attending antenatal appointments, by touching the mother's stomach, and by talking to their babies throughout the pregnancy. After birth, a father may form a strong attachment to his baby, especially if he is involved with an ill newborn's medical care while the mother is confined to her hospital bed.

Louise recalled how her husband became very attached to their baby, who lived only a few hours, while she was in bed recovering from an emergency caesarean delivery:

> Mark was with the baby the whole nine hours of his life, when I couldn't be. I had tremendous concern for him because he was so bonded with the baby. He isn't someone who expresses his emotions easily. He wasn't hysterical or anything, but I could just see it in his face.

Your Grief and the Pressure to Move On

*L*ike many fathers, you may have felt most overcome by grief immediately after the loss occurred. You may mourn intensely for a few short weeks and then make a deliberate effort to move beyond your loss. While you probably feel pulled by the need to support your partner emotionally, you may also feel an urgent desire to keep functioning and get on with your life. Withdrawing from social contacts or immersing yourself in work may provide a respite from your pain.

Joe mourned openly when his baby daughter died, but quickly felt a need to move past the loss:

> Sylvia's parents stayed with us for the first week. They were very helpful. We cried the whole week, and talked. In the process of crying and grieving, each time I had another way to look at it, why our daughter came, why she left, the growth she brought to us.
>
> The day of the cremation came. I am fuzzy about the dates. Maybe one and a half weeks after her birth. By that time I felt cried out. I made the decision to put it behind me. The day we picked up the baby's ashes was a rough day for Sylvia, but I felt a lot was behind me.

In the months that followed, there were other moments when Joe would be touched with emotion, usually when he told his story to close family or friends. But after two weeks he felt cried out, and found the worst of the pain was over for him.

Although your desire to move on may be powerful immediately after the loss, if you put aside your grief too quickly you may find it resurfaces in troubling ways long after your loss. If you are concerned about this happening to you, please see the section 'When Your Grief Is Unfinished,' toward the end of this chapter.

Your Concern for the Baby's Mother

It is often forgotten that as a father and husband you were a bystander to an event that not only took your child but also may have made you fear for your wife's safety. The loss itself may have created a high-risk medical condition, making this fear unavoidable. But even if there had been no serious medical danger, you still may have worried about your partner's well-being due to an unexpected delivery, perhaps painful or bloody, or her need for sudden sedation or surgical procedures, such as a caesarean section. You also may have been so caught up in watching and worrying about your partner's dramatic grief reactions that you neglected your own feelings.

When Hilary started bleeding in her second trimester of a twin pregnancy, she and her husband, Derek, rushed to the hospital in an unsuccessful effort to save the babies. Hilary recalled that her own medical condition was stable, but her husband doubted this from what he saw in the delivery room:

I will never forget Derek watching me. I had fetal monitors and intravenous lines attached to me. It must have been terrifying. He said to me, 'If it comes down to a choice between you and the babies, I am not going to ask what you want to do. Your life is more important.' Derek was afraid of what he saw. It looked terrible.

When the initial shock and wave of grief over the loss of the baby passed, you may have felt relief and gratitude that the baby's mother was recovering physically and was out of danger. This dual threat you experienced – for partner and child – gives you a different perspective on the loss than your wife has. If you were worried about your partner's health, let her know this, so she doesn't misinterpret your relief as meaning that you didn't care about the baby or the loss.

The Urge to be Strong

After your loss, you may have been influenced by the societal expectation that men are supposed to be 'strong' and not overly emotional. Karen Reed, a nurse who has researched the impact of pregnancy loss on fathers, has pointed out that men not only feel this initial need to be 'strong,' but also they are often so conditioned by their male roles that they cannot even let themselves cry. This expectation is reinforced if you are obliged to make practical arrangements following your loss.

Joe, whose newborn daughter died shortly after birth, described this period:

> The hospital staff came to me about permission for an autopsy. I arranged for my wife to be taken away from the maternity ward so she wouldn't be hurt more by exposure to other babies. I called our relatives with the bad news. I packed up the baby clothes and dealt with the mortuary. In the first few days, when I was taking care of the details, I had to put my grief aside.

Even when you were hurting badly, you may have tried not to look upset, in the belief that this would be best for your partner. You may have seen her falling apart emotionally and felt responsible for being the functioning member of the family while protecting her from upsetting thoughts or feelings. 'If Hilary and I were out walking and I saw a double buggy, I would try to avoid it,' explained Derek following the death of the couple's twins. 'I was trying to protect Hilary and myself.'

You may also be struggling to suppress the urge to blame the baby's mother for not providing you with the child you had successfully conceived. Even though you may know she is not at fault, your own anger, coupled with hearing her doubts about her ability to carry a child and listening to her say she feels like a 'failure,' can make you prone to blaming her.

But your efforts to spare your partner by skirting the subject of the loss and your own reactions to it can lead to misunderstanding, as she may think you are no longer sad. It is usually helpful, instead, for you to admit that you feel angry and unhappy. Your honesty won't always allay her fears, but sharing feelings and recollections can bring you closer to each other. When Derek finally admitted to Hilary that he was upset whenever he saw a double buggy, she was relieved. 'I had assumed he hadn't felt the same way I did whenever we saw twin babies,' revealed Hilary, 'when all along it was a sorrow we could have shared together.'

In contrast to the open grief of the baby's mother, you might be actively avoiding mention of your misfortune with friends and family. You may find other people are unsympathetic or embarrassed when you begin to discuss your loss, so you prefer to manage your feelings alone.

Jeff became socially withdrawn after he lost three babies to early miscarriages:

> I just didn't feel like being with people. I avoided friends with kids. I wanted to talk to certain people, but talking didn't do me any good. I would be more concerned about them. I would fill in all the clichés for them. They didn't know what to say.

Society assumes that the loss is primarily the mother's and not the father's and this probably reinforces your sense that you should not express your grief. Friends, family, and colleagues may concentrate on your partner's health and recovery and forget to ask how you are feeling. This neglect of the father's loss can reinforce your sense that you must contain or avoid your own sadness, making your mourning more difficult.

Once you become aware of this imbalance, you may find yourself responding gratefully when you are included in a friend's expression of concern. After Roger and Sarah had suffered a full-term stillbirth, Roger recalled that everybody kept asking him how his wife was coping. 'Finally a friend of mine at work asked me how *I* was doing,' he confessed. 'It really meant a lot to me.'

Maggie, who had suffered several miscarriages, noticed the same problem:

One of my friends from work came by with her husband. She had lost a baby the year before and her husband looked at my husband and said, 'How are *you* doing? Nobody asks about us!' My husband never felt he had as many outlets to talk about the loss as I had.

Like many bereaved fathers, you may have immersed yourself in work soon after your loss in an effort to do something active and constructive. You probably welcomed the chance to return to a routine and to focus on work and future goals instead of on your tragedy. 'Going back to work and my regular routine was almost a blessing,' revealed one father. 'I was able to go on with my life and think about the future, instead of dwelling on the loss or living in the past.'

Sarah Brosz Hardin, a nurse who has done research on the emotional aftermath of pregnancy loss, points out that the father's return to work may provide 'an immediate escape from grief and sadness.' But it is important to remember that this may be very different from the woman's experiences of returning to work, which usually entail constant, painful reminders of her loss.

While you may tend to be less demonstrative about your grief than your partner, you may be affected by your loss in a way that changes your entire outlook on life. Jeff explained that he returned immediately to a demanding job after his wife's third miscarriage and that grief never took over his life. But feelings about his losses remained:

Today I found out a colleague's wife is pregnant. One secretary is expecting. I say congratulations. But I wonder why this is so easy for them and not for me. I feel it's not fair.

Another father, whose premature twins died and whose wife then had two miscarriages, felt his losses had made him a more cautious person:

I am more reserved in life about things that would have excited me before. The losses put a lid on things for me. The disappointment is overwhelming. I lost my innocence.

When Your Grief Is Unfinished

The many demands placed on you as a bereaved father by the hospital, your partner, and family may allow you to grieve only briefly. You might lack socially accepted outlets for your sorrow and may feel a strong inner need to get past the pain. All these factors contribute to the likelihood that your mourning will be cut short to some degree.

Yet, for many fathers, grief does not end quickly. You may have expressed your feelings of loss only partially, and then let them become submerged as your energies were diverted into work and taking care of the baby's mother. Your grief may take the form of anger that your basic assumptions about having a family have been upset. You may find yourself becoming jealous and resentful of friends and family who are in the process of having babies or raising small children. Your loss can even leave you doubting your ability to set and achieve important goals in your life.

Feelings of mourning may re-emerge with anniversaries of the birth or loss, or during holidays and family gatherings, often taking you by surprise. While upsetting, this resurgence of memories and feelings about your pregnancy loss can enable you to continue the mourning process that was left unfinished. Try to take the opportunity to talk with your partner, family, friends, a member of the clergy, or a psychotherapist. Joining a pregnancy loss support group such as SANDS can help give expression to your frustration and sorrow. One bereaved father described how verbalizing his feelings helped him:

> I've never had to grieve before. I've had grandparents pass away. But that's different – it's part of life to grow old and get sick and die. But not a baby. Our baby's death was so unfair. And this loss was so close to us – so personal. Talking enabled me to express the grief and come to terms with it. It made me a better person.

What Can Help Bereaved Fathers

*L*ike most bereaved fathers, you probably feel you must be 'strong' for your family and may be denying yourself the chance to demonstrate your sorrow openly and effectively. Immediately after the pregnancy loss occurs, you may have many burdens to carry, such as responsibility for practical but upsetting arrangements related to the loss, and worry about the baby's mother, all of which may put your grief on hold. But if you do not express your grief now it can re-emerge in destructive ways later.

Here are some suggestions that can enable you to deal with the demands placed on you without repressing your own grief response:

- Include your partner in decisions about the baby if she is able to participate. This will help both of you feel connected to each other as well as to your child.

- You may have to appear strong at times, but try to give yourself time for your feelings as well, with your partner, with a loved one, or alone.

- If you were worried about your partner's health, let her know so she doesn't misinterpret your relief at her recovery to mean you did not care about the baby.

- You may find your return to work to be a welcome relief from constant sadness over the loss. Although you are entitled to that relief, consider setting aside a limited time during each week to recall, write about, or talk about the loss. Though difficult, expressing your grief can allow you to resolve your pain.

CHAPTER 4

PREGNANCY LOSS AND YOUR RELATIONSHIP: GRIEVING TOGETHER AND APART

I don't remember our sex life being different after the loss. Our sex life was good before and after. There was no change really.

MARK

When we talked about the loss we got into trouble because we would fight. We just got on each other's nerves over other things, too.

LISA

I felt like someone had pulled a plug. We were both so drained.

DEREK

Your pregnancy loss forces you and your partner to grapple with a serious crisis, perhaps the first you have ever shared. Your relationship is put to a test that can either draw you together or drive you apart. If you are fortunate, family and friends are there to help, but more likely you have been left to manage your devastation with little outside support. Even the most compassionate friends and relatives might not continue to reach out and sustain you for nearly as long as you need them. Aware of this lack of understanding, you and your partner may isolate yourselves and turn to each other as your primary – or only – source of comfort.

Your Relationship During the Crisis

During and after the immediate crisis of your loss, you and your partner probably felt close to one another because of the shared trauma. Together you lived through the anxiety, fear, emergency medical care, and ultimately the loss of your baby.

Having shared this ordeal, it is likely that you turned to one another for solace, each of you feeling grateful for the physical and emotional presence of the other. 'There was this sense that we've gone through this experience together,' Jeff said after his wife's third miscarriage. 'There was this very strong feeling that at least we had each other and should hold on to that.'

When Maggie and Bert's premature baby daughter died, Maggie was grateful that they both stayed at home and grieved together at first:

> Bert had wanted the baby very badly, and he took her death very hard. He couldn't share my physical pain, but as much as he could share without actually carrying the baby, he was there. His being home with me for a few days helped us to be loving together and be miserable together. He was very supportive.

You may each take turns mourning and supporting one another immediately after your pregnancy loss. When one of you is most out of control, the other holds together and is the consoler, and then your roles switch. 'I think it was too much for both of us to fall apart,' one bereaved father remarked. 'I was relieved that my wife was more in control when I went to pieces. Then I took the ball when she was grieving.'

A bereaved mother often finds she is still nonfunctional during the first few weeks after a loss. She may cry constantly, have insomnia and nightmares, and feel unable to get out of bed. Although the baby's father is probably back at work, perhaps after only a few days' leave, he may continue to care for her and help her, sometimes in thoughtful, touching ways.

Lisa credited her husband for gently prodding her out of her lethargy after their newborn baby died:

> After our loss, I just vegetated in front of the TV. Adam was great. He finally wrote me lists. 'Do two things on this list today,' he said. Then the next day he said, 'Do three things on this list.' Eventually I could do things and get out of the house.

Sometimes the baby's father responds to the mother's continuing depression by sympathetically insisting that she engage in an enjoyable activity, whether an exercise class, a regular outing to the cinema, or a hobby. As long as he is also respectful of her need to grieve, this type of persuasion can work very well.

Months after her premature son died, Louise refused to go out of the house at all, except to work. Her husband became impatient and worried until he hit on an idea. He knew Louise had always enjoyed singing, and before losing her baby, she had planned to join a choral group. She remembered the night her husband literally dragged her to one of their rehearsals:

> Outside in the hall I heard them singing and said to by husband, 'I'm not that good. Please don't make me go in.' But with his encouragement, I not only went in, but I sang with that group for two years and it was very therapeutic.

After the initial crisis has passed, bereaved parents may become acutely aware of the differences in their grieving. By this time their families probably expect them to be getting on with their lives. Visits and phone calls from friends are infrequent or stop. The baby's father is back to his work routine and, although he may still be grieving, he might not want to express his feelings openly or might not even be aware of them. Yet the mother is most likely still in active mourning, whether she is at home or back at work, and she may continue to grieve openly for many months.

This is when a bereaved mother can begin to find the baby's father unfeeling and unsupportive, while he begins to tire of her extreme emotions and wonder if she will ever get better. And this is when incongruent grief – the very different courses mourning can follow – begins to take its toll.

Incongruent Grief

He wondered why I wasn't feeling better; I wondered why he wasn't feeling worse.

SYLVIA

The differing intensity and duration of mourning a mother and father may experience can create stress in your relationship, especially if you don't realize that such incongruent grief is quite common. Instead, you may feel angry and critical of your partner for grieving differently.

Deep fears usually lie at the root of this conflict. A bereaved father can become convinced that something is seriously wrong with his continually grieving wife. She then feels betrayed by the one person she had relied on to understand her, comfort her, and share in the loss.

A grieving mother may misinterpret her husband's faster recovery and contained emotions as lack of love for the baby and may mistake his relief at her own physical recovery for lack of sorrow about the loss. Perhaps the baby's father believes he should suppress his grief to remain functional so he can help her. As misunderstanding builds, marital trust is shaken.

Adam's helplessness and frustration grew as he tried, unsuccessfully, to make Louise feel better after their newborn daughter's death:

> I tried to say things which I thought were comforting, and it turned out they had the opposite effect. It was also difficult for Louise to understand what a father would feel under these circumstances, especially since my grief seemed shorter.

Anger, guilt, and attempts to place blame for the loss are distressing aspects of bereavement. It is natural for you sometimes to direct these negative feelings toward your partner. If your relationship is strong and you realize that anger is part of your grief, you can tolerate these outbursts and actually help each other. Roger recalled how he and his wife both broke down and yet depended on one another through the delivery of their stillborn son:

> When I first found out, I started punching the pillow on the hospital bed and kept sobbing, 'Why? Why?' over and over. I was so angry and out of control. But just being with each other physically at first, literally clinging to each other, was helpful. We knew we could do this in front of each other and it would be okay.

But not all partners can tolerate such anger. You may feel personally attacked by your partner's outrage and may sense that one of you is blaming the other for causing the tragedy. Or you may find that anger comes out in other areas so that issues that had not been problematic before suddenly become the focus of conflict.

One couple who hardly ever argued prior to their loss found themselves in constant conflict afterward:

> We had so much anger toward each other. I was so angry I needed to hit pillows and throw things and beat the bed. I was angry about his working with a female executive at his office. I really had no reason to be jealous of her, but I was. When we talked we got into trouble because we would fight. We just got on each other's nerves.

A bereaved father may avoid bringing up the pregnancy loss with his partner after his own initial upset is over. He may feel that discussing the loss will make her more depressed, or he may be seeking relief from his own painful memories. 'As time went on, it got hard to talk,' explained Derek. 'I didn't like to see my wife upset. I wanted to talk about other things.'

But a husband's avoidance of the topic can backfire, because his wife may truly need to talk about their baby, her sadness, or her jealousy each time she sees a pregnant woman or a new mother. She may experience her husband's reluctance to talk about the baby as emotional abandonment, especially if she has no one else to turn to. Hilary, Derek's wife, found that her need to talk about their twins who died and his need not to talk eventually hurt both of them:

> In the beginning we talked about the babies, the grief, and when to try to get pregnant again. But then Derek said, 'I want to talk about the loss but not all the time.' I said, 'If I can't talk to you, who can I talk to?' We both understood each other but couldn't help each other.

When you feel the need to talk about the loss either more or less than your partner, you may find it helpful to set aside a specific and limited time each day, or later on once a week, to talk about the baby together. In this way you can share your thoughts and feelings with each other without worrying that grief will become an all-consuming preoccupation or that your needs will not be respected. 'I tried not to talk as much about the loss,' explained Hilary, when she and her husband reached this compromise. 'If he had a decent day, talking could crash it in. And because of our arrangement, I felt he tried to listen to me more.'

Incongruent grief can cause serious problems when your grief reaction is so different from your partner's you can no longer empathize with one another. You may stop wanting or even trying to talk to your partner and may end up feeling angry, misunderstood, and emotionally distant.

Amelia found it increasingly difficult to cope with the news of friends' and colleagues' pregnancies after her own losses. She also got more and more upset when her husband neither shared nor understood her feelings:

> I was consumed by jealousy and bitterness. And worse than that for me was that Charles didn't seem to feel the same anger and resentment I did. I felt he didn't support or understand my rage. I desperately needed someone to talk to about my feelings each time I heard about someone else getting pregnant, but Charles just didn't seem to share my feelings and I couldn't talk to him easily.

If these sharp differences in a couple's grief responses are not understood, they can lead to a total communication breakdown. As time goes on, the bereaved father may want his life to get back to normal and might blame his wife's continuing distress for the fact that they no longer enjoy shared activities or one another. 'I was screaming and having hysterical fits while Joe was contained and wanted to get on with things,' revealed Sylvia. 'He got tired of my being so emotional. Both of us felt justified in our feelings and believed the other was 'wrong.''

Joe felt that their different grief reactions got to the point where mistrust, anger, and anxiety began to take over their marriage:

> I told Sylvia that I had heard enough crying, that I thought we were getting better. Her reaction was to clam up. Then, when I tried to talk about the baby, she told me that I didn't really want to hear about it and she wouldn't let me bring up the subject, which left me really angry.
>
> Sometimes she would say she missed the baby, or felt defective as a woman, and I would tell her I didn't know she was feeling that way. Then she would snap that she felt this way all the time. It made me feel so out of touch. There were times when I thought Sylvia would never get better.

If you reach this kind of serious but common impasse in trust and communication, it is vital to try to talk to your partner and re-establish contact. By making time to sit down together and taking turns talking to each other, your feelings and worries can be aired and explored. This may enable you to learn that each of you is pulling away from the other due to hurt and fear, not from lack of love for each other or the baby. As your misunderstandings clear, mutual respect and support can again become possible. If you are having difficulty doing this, seek outside help. Once you have re-established communication with each other, you may be greatly relieved to discover that although your reactions are very different, they are entirely understandable.

Your Grief and Sexuality

After the miscarriage I didn't have a problem with having sex at all. It was so comforting, so exciting. We had missed each other so much.

LOUISE

I didn't want to be touched. Sex felt forced. I was sad because the loss had taken the joy out of sex as well as out of pregnancy and childbearing.

SYLVIA

Pregnancy loss can affect every aspect of your marriage, including your sexual relationship. Your reaction to resuming sex will be highly individual and may be quite different from your partner's. Perhaps you and your partner are one of the few couples whose loss has increased your physical need for one another. For you, sex is a source of comfort and pleasure, a way of expressing the closeness you feel from having endured and helped one another through your tragedy. 'We had always been very much in love,' recalled Adam, 'and, if anything, our tragedy made us realize how lucky we were to have each other, both physically and emotionally.'

But for most parents, resuming sexual relations after a pregnancy loss is highly charged. Although your doctor may have insisted on a specific period of abstinence, these medical restrictions do not take into account the complicated feelings about sex you may have following your loss. Your reactions to the loss, sex, birth control, and conceiving again can become interrelated and extremely upsetting after your pregnancy ends.

Couples may follow the standard medical recommendation of waiting four to six weeks after a loss before resuming sexual relations. Doctors suggest this period to give the cervix time to close and heal, limiting the chance of uterine infection or other physical damage. A period of abstinence is also recommended following a caesarean section if labour began before the surgery. Doctors urge couples to wait so the uterus can return to its original size and the lining has time to shed and heal, giving any subsequent pregnancy the best possible chance of implanting properly. If there was an episiotomy, it, too, must have sufficient time to heal to prevent tearing or other damage during intercourse.

Once you have abstained the requisite number of weeks and are free to resume sexual relations, you may discover that sex vividly reminds you of the pregnancy that ended tragically. Thoughts about the loss may resurface when you make love as you are reminded of the last pregnancy you conceived. You might urgently wish to become pregnant again, while your partner may be terrified at the prospect of another pregnancy. These memories and preoccupations can make you lose your sexual desire.

Maggie found that both she and her husband approached sex gingerly after losing their premature baby. 'It brought out a lot of feelings,' she recalled. 'Having sex was like getting my period after the loss – I felt sad that I wasn't pregnant anymore. Sex also had the danger of becoming a chore, an obligation. The loss took away all the spontaneity.'

A husband may worry about physically hurting his wife during intercourse, as he thinks she may be sore after childbirth, an episiotomy, a

D&C, or other surgery. His concern about her physical tenderness may be tied in with guilt for having conceived the pregnancy that put her through the pain and grief of a loss. Taken together, these feelings can make him reluctant to approach her sexually.

Sarah and Roger experienced this problem after their first child was stillborn. 'First Roger was afraid of hurting me, as I was sore from the episiotomy for some time after the loss,' Sarah explained. 'Then he became afraid to have sex, even though the doctor said it was okay.'

Even the use of birth control, which is usually a straightforward matter, can be depressing after a pregnancy loss. You and your partner may realize you need time to heal emotionally before conceiving again; but because you have lost the baby you wanted so much, deciding not to conceive a child every time you make love can be very distressing.

Jeff felt there was a lot of sadness around the use of birth control after he and his wife had suffered three miscarriages:

> Birth control became a loaded issue. We needed some time before attempting another pregnancy in addition to the physical wait after the D&C. But the idea of sex with a contraceptive felt horrible. Sometimes I couldn't escape the focus, and it bothered my wife all the time. It interfered with our sexual pleasure a lot.

Even though it might be difficult to talk about sex, it is important for you and your partner to be frank with one another about your readiness to resume relations, as well as your readiness to plan another pregnancy. Although birth control can be hard to contemplate initially, continue to use it until you feel prepared for another pregnancy. Gradually, as each of you gets better emotionally, sexual pleasure will probably return, and the sad associations between birth control and the pregnancy loss will lessen.

You may be like some bereaved parents who lose all sexual interest after a pregnancy loss, sometimes for a long time. You may feel extremely vulnerable after losing your baby, and may not want to be intimate out of a need for self-protection. You may feel cheated because sex is not giving you what you truly want, which is not just physical pleasure but a healthy baby as well. Tensions in your relationship, including mistrust and resentment over the differing ways you and your partner cope with the loss, can also contribute to your lack of interest in sex.

When you feel ready to have another baby, and resume sexual relations, sex may again go 'on hold' once you conceive. Although doctors rarely consider sex to cause pregnancy loss, they may recommend that if you have had a certain kind of loss you should abstain from intercourse as an extra precaution. Some couples take this precaution upon themselves because it makes them feel they are doing something to protect the pregnancy. But this can mean a long period of sexual abstinence, and serious marital strain.

Sylvia's aversion to sex continued for several months after her newborn daughter died, and once she was pregnant again:

> I didn't want to be touched. I felt physically damaged, bruised, hurt. I bled for a long time. I leaked milk and had a large episiotomy. I turned into myself. It took me a long time to feel physically better. I didn't want sexual contact for six months. I wanted to be left alone, to curl up in the fetal position in a blanket.
>
> In March we wanted to try to become pregnant again. That was the only reason for having sex; there was no pleasure in it. These feelings persisted until I became pregnant again. Then I wanted to be left alone with this new baby. I needed my body for myself. It was even hard to share it with the baby, let alone with my husband.

While a period of sexual abstinence sometimes cannot be avoided after a loss, you and your partner may pay a price for any long hiatus in your sexual relationship. Sexual tensions can add significantly to the marital stress brought on by bereavement. Your partner may not always agree that abstinence after a pregnancy loss is a wise or necessary choice. As one father remarked, 'We were much too cautious, and it wouldn't have made a difference in our particular case. Abstaining created a strain.'

It is important for you to talk honestly about your sexual needs to prevent resentment from building after a loss or during a subsequent pregnancy. Perhaps you can work out ways to give and receive sexual pleasure without intercourse, so that sexual frustrations do not add to the other pressures you are experiencing. Oral sex and mutual masturbation can be pleasurable ways to reduce sexual tensions; however, a pregnant woman's partner should avoid blowing air into the vagina, as this could introduce a potentially dangerous air bubble into a maternal blood vessel.

Some women must avoid climaxes during a precarious pregnancy because orgasms can stimulate dangerous uterine contractions. But some degree of physical intimacy is still possible. 'Even when I chose not to have a climax,' admitted one woman about the pregnancy that followed her miscarriages, 'it made me feel close to my husband and better about our sex life if I at least helped him achieve an orgasm.'

If you find your sexual needs are different from your partner's after your loss, especially if your relationship is stressed in other ways, you may benefit greatly from outside support or professional help. You may even be harbouring unrealistic fears that sexual intercourse contributed to your pregnancy loss. Learning that sexual difficulties during bereavement are common can help you open communication and meet your partner halfway.

You and your partner may decide you need a period of relaxed sexual relations after suffering your pregnancy loss and may delay your plans to conceive because of this. You may feel you have gone through pain and heartache from your loss and are anxious about whether the next child you conceive will be born healthy. You may not want to add to these difficulties by depriving yourself of the intimacy and comfort of sexual pleasure.

Louise spent two months in and out of the hospital trying to save her pregnancy, without success and with tremendous strains on her sex life.

> It was important that I not have any orgasms as well as not having intercourse. The doctor wouldn't allow any uterine contractions. It was driving me crazy not to have sex. It became a real joke. When I was in the hospital, I remember saying to my doctor, 'I can't work, I can't take care of my family, I can't have sex. What can I do? Can I at least take some vitamins?'

I worry about the next pregnancy because it will mean no sexual intercourse. It's a reason for me to postpone it.

How Pregnancy Loss Can Change Your Relationship

Having endured a pregnancy loss, you and your partner may find your relationship has been permanently changed. As you each live through your loss and grief, you may feel estranged from your partner because of your differing responses to the loss. You may even experience grave doubts about whether you can count on either yourself or your partner to pull through the ordeal intact and committed to the relationship.

Yet, like many couples, you and your partner may not only pull through but also discover your relationship has been strengthened through the tragedy you endured together. You may uncover resilience and resolution in yourself and in your spouse that you never experienced before. You can feel you have gained a richer understanding of one another, both as individuals and as partners.

Eric and Annette had tried to conceive a baby for four years before finally achieving pregnancy. When the baby stopped growing eight weeks into the pregnancy, Eric was moved by the way Annette prepared herself for a D&C:

> This was one of the worst experiences of Annette's life. She had wanted to be pregnant for so long, and then to lose the baby – it was unimaginable. I remember so clearly the way she set her alarm clock and got up the day of the D&C. She went to the hospital and came home with a manner of acceptance I was unprepared to see. I was incredibly impressed by her bravery.

If you and your partner can convey caring for one another in your bereavement in spite of feeling vulnerable or at times misunderstood, you may emerge with a deep sense of faith in your relationship. You will have passed through a crucible of sorrow that leaves you confident that you can face and survive other trials you will inevitably encounter.

Karen believed her five miscarriages affected her marriage profoundly:

> I think there is a certain celebration in our relationship because we have been through these losses but are still so close and caring. It's made the good times better and the bad times bearable. Our marriage was tested over and over again, so now we know we will always be there for each other.

If you have other children, you may find that the shared tragedy has left you with a sense of unity and understanding that equips you to handle crises of parenthood as nothing else in your experience has done. When your child is ill or in need, you and your partner may know instantly where your priorities lie and can mobilize yourselves with strength and clarity of purpose.

One husband, whose wife had suffered four miscarriages, arranged for a colleague to conclude a vital business deal instead, because he wanted to stay with his infant daughter who required emergency hospitalization. 'My partners told me it would be impossible to find a last-minute replacement,' he recalled, 'but I found a way to close the deal legally without actually being there. It was more important for me to be with my family.'

Through the tragedy of their loss, parents often find they know their priorities and have learned how to pull together to protect what is most important to them. Ellen told how her husband had joined her in the hospital recovery room with their sobbing two-year-old who was just out of surgery, in spite of hospital regulations that permitted only one parent at a time. 'His coming in against the rules reminded me of his determination when he stayed in my hospital room all night after my miscarriage,' she explained.

But not all couples fare so well after a pregnancy loss, and for some, the crisis of a loss takes a serious toll on their relationship. Even if your relationship is good, you may temporarily criticize or feel angry with your spouse after your loss. And if your relationship had tensions, conflicts, or unaired resentments before the loss, your grief can trigger cruel attacks, accusations of blame, or complete withdrawal.

Sometimes relationships do break up after a pregnancy loss. Disappointments with each other that were kept in check when your life together was stable can become intolerable in a crisis. And when your relationship is tested by tragedy, one or both of you may be devastated when the other fails to come through with needed solace and support. This happened to Julia and her ex-husband:

> My first husband and I were totally thrown apart by the miscarriage. There was no support at all from him. I went in for a D&C and he refused to drive me to the hospital. I was so hysterical about this, the doctor had to tranquilize me. I could hear the nurses talking about why my husband wasn't with me. When I woke up from the anaesthetic, I woke up crying. At first I thought I must be in physical pain, but then I realized I was distraught because I needed my husband with me so much, and he wasn't there. When I went home my husband said, 'Everyone has D&Cs. It's no big deal.' That was the beginning of the end.

Your relationship may dissolve after your loss because you see one another at your most needy and vulnerable and may not like what you see. One woman was engaged to be married when she unexpectedly became pregnant and then miscarried. Shortly afterward, her fiancé left her:

> He said I was no longer the person he knew before the miscarriage. He said when he met me I was strong and beautiful. And here I was lying in the fetal position, weeping. Now I think the breakup was for the best. If it hadn't been the miscarriage, he would have left me at some other crisis. I would have been alone for the hard times.

If your relationship is in serious trouble after your loss, you and your partner must deal with two cataclysmic events – pregnancy loss and potential separation – simultaneously. You need to begin sorting out your feelings about the loss and one another as quickly as possible. Try to have open discussions allotting equal time for each of you to express your concerns, and try to listen patiently to each other's reactions to the loss. This dialogue can help your mutual and individual adjustments following your loss, whether you ultimately decide to stay together or to separate.

If you cannot begin to talk with each other openly and honestly, or if your individual feelings are still too hurtful to each other, a support group or sessions with a counsellor skilled in bereavement issues can be especially beneficial.

Although pregnancy loss can strain marital relationships, many couples ultimately remain committed to their union and family. They may even emerge with a special appreciation for one another. Paula found this to be so after losing a baby following a medical crisis in her pregnancy:

> My husband and I were very close anyway, but the loss brought us closer. Losing the baby reinforced our wonder at the next child and confirmed our wanting to have the next child. We never again took for granted what happens in pregnancy.

What Can Help You Grieve Individually and Together

Your pregnancy loss and grief have probably touched every aspect of your relationship. You and your partner may be brought closer, and your commitment to each other strengthened, as a result of surviving the tragedy together. But your relationship can also be stressed by incongruent grief, especially if each of you thinks the other is 'wrong' for reacting differently to the loss. Criticism is conveyed and resentment sets in. You may each feel misunderstood, if not betrayed, at a time when you are in critical need of the other's support.

While grief must run its course, the stresses of incongruent grief can be alleviated. It is important to realize that each of you will experience grief in a unique way. A mother's grief may well be more intense and prolonged, while the baby's father may need help in finding ways to express his underlying sadness.

You can help each other by listening to one another's feelings without judgment and without expecting to feel exactly the same way. You may also benefit from psychotherapy or other outside help, such as a pregnancy loss support group like SANDS which can validate your and your partner's unique responses to the loss while helping you share and resolve unfinished grief together.

Here are some suggestions to help you weather the difficult days and weeks ahead:

- Give yourself time to grieve, on your own and with your partner. Expect to need support from others in addition to your mate, who is emotionally depleted, too. It is essential to grieve your loss because unexpressed grief can emerge later as depression, anxiety, anger, or marital stress.
- Expect your grief response to be different from your partner's. Frankly share your feelings and needs, but do not expect your partner to react the same way. Be respectful of your partner's differing needs, and try to be understanding without judging one another.
- You may experience changes in sexual desire that differ from your partner's reactions. Share your sexual feelings and needs frankly, and try to be sensitive to each other. It is best not to try to conceive again until both you and your partner feel ready. Any sexual problems usually improve as mourning progresses.
- If serious problems develop in your relationship after your pregnancy loss, understand that grief has stressed your union and has made other issues more evident during the crisis. Couple or individual psychotherapy can help you sort out problems due to grief from other underlying problems.
- Remember that it takes time to grieve and that gradually the pain will lessen. You will always remember your baby, but you will once again experience pleasure and hope for the future. Surviving the tragedy of pregnancy loss with your partner can give you a new appreciation for one another and for what is most important to you.

SECTION II
....

PREGNANCY LOSS EXAMINED

With the misfortune of your pregnancy loss, you and your partner have temporarily lost the dream of becoming parents or of providing a sibling for your other children. No matter what type of loss you experienced, you share with other bereaved parents a bond of sorrow, endurance, and hope as you live through your tragedy and begin to build a future after your loss. Yet each loss remains unique, with its own medical implications and emotional impact.

The issues you faced were quite different if you suffered a stillbirth or newborn death rather than a loss early in the pregnancy. You had to decide whether to name your baby, or to say goodbye with formal rituals. If your loss occurred in the first three months, or trimester, you may have been spared some of these difficult decisions, but loved ones, doctors, and clergy may have been less likely to acknowledge your sorrow and help you mourn.

The medical concerns that now confront you also depend on the kind of pregnancy loss you suffered. If you experienced consecutive miscarriages, you are probably anxious about what caused them and what treatments are available to you. If your baby died from a cord accident in the womb or from birth defects, you must grapple with the heightened uneasiness an unpreventable misfortune brings to any subsequent pregnancy.

Parents face a particularly lonely and painful experience if antenatal diagnosis indicated a severe problem with the baby and they decided to terminate their pregnancy. And if a loss occurred toward the end of the mother's most fertile years, both parents may be worried about never having another successful pregnancy, a fear that couples in their twenties probably won't share.

Nearly one third of all conceptions end in some type of natural pregnancy loss, with almost 80 percent of all losses occurring in the first three months of pregnancy, about 14 percent in the second trimester, and approximately 6 percent in the third. Sadly, if you have experienced more than one previous loss, you are at increased risk of suffering another.

But statistics mean very little when you have lost your baby. 'No matter what the chances are,' said one woman, 'if it happens to you, it happens 100 percent.' And in spite of the frequency of pregnancy loss, you may have difficulty finding compassionate support for your grief. You may bear the additional burden of having to initiate conversations with your doctor on potential treatments to safeguard future pregnancies.

This section, 'Pregnancy Loss Examined,' discusses the different emotional and medical issues associated with early losses, stillbirth, and newborn death, as well as losses caused by crisis pregnancies and abortions following prenatal testing. By understanding the symptoms, causes, treatments, and emotional impact associated with your loss, you can begin to gain a perspective on your problem and its eventual resolution.

CHAPTER 5

EARLY LOSSES

I felt devastated after my second miscarriage. From childhood, a little girl is taught she will grow up to be a bride and a mother. Motherhood is revered. This dream of having a baby is from childhood. It was the dream that was being wiped out.

AMY

A first-trimester loss is a silent loss, one that often goes unacknowledged by outsiders who fail to recognize the agonizing emptiness it leaves behind. When you lose a baby early in the pregnancy, you may have to deal with a lack of concrete memories about the pregnancy or your baby and the absence of any ritual to mark this sad event.

You may feel some small comfort in learning that you are not alone, since most pregnancy losses occur during the first three months of pregnancy. Miscarriages account for almost 95 percent of all early losses up to twenty-four weeks' gestation, after which they are considered to be live births or stillbirths. Ectopic pregnancies, in which implantation occurs outside the uterus, make up about 4 percent of the total. The remaining 1 percent of early losses consists of rare forms of pregnancy loss, such as molar pregnancies, in which fertilization occurs but there is no fetus and the placenta rapidly develops into a ball of cells which can become malignant in a very small percentage of women.

An early loss ends the pregnancy just as it is beginning, only weeks or even days after you first realized you and your partner were going to be parents. Your joyous expectations were suddenly turned to grief, and the pregnancy, which ended so early, may now seem completely unreal.

Issues Common to All Early Losses

Although a woman's hormones shift immediately and dramatically to support a new pregnancy, the changes in her body during the first few weeks after conception are subtle and personal. She may feel nauseous and her breasts may be tender, but the pregnancy is still a secret, locked invisibly inside her body. Friends and family cannot see any change in her body until much later in the pregnancy, and she may wish to keep her secret a while longer, savouring it with her partner. Both parents may also feel superstitious about telling anyone about the pregnancy too soon, afraid that their joy may become jinxed.

When a pregnancy ends early in the first trimester, most mothers immediately feel shocked and bereft, but the impact on fathers is often delayed. Even fathers who share in pregnancy tests, visits to the GP, and early scans, can have a difficult time absorbing the reality of a pregnancy that ends just as it is beginning. Eric admitted that his wife's first-trimester loss only seemed real to him after it was over. 'It was something I hadn't felt part of or emotional about and suddenly I was crying about it for days,' he confessed. 'It amazed me that this was how and when I knew I cared about the pregnancy – only once it was over.'

The lack of tangible reminders of your pregnancy can keep each of you from grieving properly. Even the smallest keepsake can help. Annette cherished her scan photographs of the first-trimester pregnancy she eventually miscarried. Although she didn't look at the pictures often, it was comforting to have them tucked away. In a subsequent, healthy pregnancy, another scan reawakened feelings about the image of the tiny baby she never knew:

> We learned so much about this current pregnancy after the scans and amniocentesis – that we're expecting twins and that they are girls. I kept looking at them moving around on the ultrasound screen and kept wondering to myself, 'Who was that first child? Who was that baby we lost?'

Tangible reminders of a pregnancy that ended in the first trimester can also help you and your partner release feelings of disappointment and grief. After Natalie's third loss, she went home to her living room, where she had a picture from the scan and some congratulation cards from friends and family. 'I was so upset, I took them off the mantelpiece,' she explained, 'and threw them all out.'

You may be feeling isolated and alone after your early loss, especially if your friends and family do not acknowledge how upset you are. They may not have been aware of your pregnancy until the loss occurred, forcing them to absorb both pieces of news at once and leaving them little time to develop a sense of what the events mean to you and your partner.

Few people offer enough sympathy after an early loss because they do not comprehend its impact. This leaves both you and your partner without support when you most need others to talk with you and to listen compassionately. Eric withdrew from people when he felt they didn't realize how much his wife's miscarriage affected him:

> When people didn't seem to understand, it became a good reason to shut up about the loss and not talk about it anymore. I think people would have understood more easily if they could have seen the pregnancy. People tend to dismiss it if it is an early loss.

Well-intentioned people may utter platitudes such as 'It was only an early loss,' or 'It happened for the best,' in an attempt to reassure both you and themselves. They may also assume that because the loss occurred so early, you should recover quickly and have another child right away. But pregnancy losses should be acknowledged and mourned, and these comments only make you feel your sadness is somehow inappropriate because the pregnancy was so brief.

As time passes and you start to feel better, you may be confused if, without warning, you suddenly feel worse again. Emotional reactions can be triggered by the onset of the woman's menstrual cycle after an early loss, as well as the arrival of her subsequent periods or the baby's due date. In particular, the first period after an early loss reiterates the failed pregnancy, but also indicates that the woman's body is returning to a normal cycle, preparing itself for another possible pregnancy.

Annette was ecstatic about getting her first period after the loss and even called her husband at work to tell him the news. 'It was the best thing since the loss,' she remembered. 'I took it as a sign that my body was back in working order. But every period after that I felt was a sorrow, because it reminded me I wasn't pregnant anymore or again.'

Your early pregnancy loss may affect you in ways you did not expect, especially if you have had more than one loss. You may be preoccupied about undergoing medical tests before you plan another pregnancy, or you may feel depressed far longer than you anticipated. 'I'm normally a happy, productive person who loves life,' professed Karen, 'and I resent all this grieving and emotional upheaval following each of my losses.'

No matter what type of early loss you suffered, you will need time as you recover emotionally and support as you pursue your next pregnancy. Consider joining a support group or making an appointment with a psychotherapist if you feel the need.

You may also find yourself searching for some meaning to your tragedy, a way of accepting that your baby's presence, no matter how brief, was life-affirming. As Stuart, whose wife suffered three first-trimester miscarriages, said:

> It seems to me we have two choices: one is to become withdrawn and bitter and angry and the other is to integrate this experience into our lives so it leaves a positive legacy. As hard as it sometimes is, we are trying to make that positive choice.

Experiencing a Miscarriage

My wife, Virginia, suffered two miscarriages in one six-month period, one in the spring and the next one in September. Nine months later we found out Virginia was pregnant again.

We went for a scan and there on the monitor was the heartbeat! It was so wonderful to have the pregnancy documented that way. The doctor said that everything looked fine, that everything was great and perfect.

Virginia was still nervous and afraid because of her other losses, but she was so happy. The doctor said she could come back anytime she needed to be reassured about the pregnancy. That made us both feel better.

A few days later it was our son's birthday and we would normally have had a party for him in our garden. But Virginia was trying to reduce stress in our lives, so we held the party in a nearby hall. We came home from the party and our son was opening his presents when Virginia said she had to go to the bathroom. When she came back she told me she was bleeding quite heavily. We had a scan the next day. The doctor confirmed that the baby had died. We were devastated.

PATRICK

Miscarriage is an unexpected and disheartening experience. The statistics on miscarriage in general, and for older parents in particular, are on a tragic rising trajectory. This is due in part to the increase in late childbearing in our society, which augments the rate of all pregnancy losses each year. In more than half of all miscarriages a cause cannot be determined, which can add to parents' uncertainty and anxiety about planning future pregnancies.

Symptoms and Diagnosis of a Miscarriage

Signs of a miscarriage can vary from one pregnancy loss to another, even in the same mother, making it hard to recognize potentially serious symptoms. Sometimes all the outward signals are present, such as bleeding, cramping, or the loss of nausea and other pregnancy symptoms, but often only one sign appears as a single, ambiguous warning.

Although vaginal bleeding is a symptom in many early losses, bleeding occurs in more than 30 percent of all pregnancies in the first trimester. Half of these bleeding episodes resolve, and the pregnancies continue normally, so it is often difficult to determine when concern should become alarm.

Cramping in the early months of healthy pregnancies is also common, making it hard to know when the pain has moved across the dangerous borderline into the strong, rhythmic uterine contractions that often accompany a miscarriage. Ellen recalled waking up in the middle of the night with what felt like severe period pains during her first pregnancy:

> There was no blood, so I just lay in bed for a while wondering what I should do next. I didn't understand what was happening, but for some reason the word 'labour' came to mind, even though I'd never had a baby before. The pains were becoming stronger and more rhythmical, and I was quite frightened. I finally woke up my husband and we called my doctor, who felt I was probably losing the baby.

Miscarriages can also occur without the common symptoms of bleeding and cramping pains. Since the mother cannot feel the baby's movements early in the pregnancy, she is equally unaware when they stop. It may be weeks after the baby died before her body attempts to expel the pregnancy with uterine contractions and bleeding. If the pregnancy had been progressing nicely, she may be totally unprepared to discover she has experienced a loss.

A doctor can confirm an early miscarriage by several means. If the pregnancy is beyond eleven weeks, listening for the heartbeat with an instrument called a sonicaid is the first step. If no heartbeat is found, the doctor does both an internal and an external examination to see if there is any uterine or cervical change, or if any elements of the pregnancy have passed into the vagina. Tests that determine the amount of pregnancy hormones in the mother's bloodstream are accurate but can take up to forty-eight hours for final results, a long time for anxious parents to wait.

The most conclusive and immediate test is a scan, so the doctor can visualize and evaluate the condition of the womb, embryonic sac, and baby. Because a healthy, developing baby is visible on an ultrasound screen as early as eight to nine weeks in gestation, even earlier if a vaginal scan is used, its absence is equally clear.

Treating a Miscarriage

Your doctor may have recommended bed rest for miscarriage symptoms, even though no scientific studies have established bed rest as an effective treatment for early spontaneous losses. Once you began to miscarry in the first trimester, you probably lost the pregnancy whether or not you stayed in bed.

If a doctor finds that all the products of the pregnancy have been expelled – baby, sac, placenta, and uterine lining – she may suggest that the patient go home, rest for a few days, and try to conceive again once she has a couple of normal menstrual cycles. If some elements of the pregnancy remain in the uterus, the doctor either recommends that the woman wait until everything is expelled naturally, or else the doctor performs a dilatation and curettage, known as a D&C, to remove the remaining material.

Since a D&C is considered an elective procedure and is not usually an emergency, a woman may have to wait for treatment, which can be both frightening and physically painful. The procedure takes about twenty minutes, followed by an hour or so in the recovery room to make sure the woman's pulse, blood pressure, respiratory rate, and temperature are stable before she is discharged. Vaginal bleeding that tapers off over several days is common after a D&C.

Causes of Miscarriage

Once the immediate trauma of the miscarriage is behind you, you may begin wondering why the pregnancy ended so early. You may be afraid to plan another pregnancy without some medical answers, especially if you have suffered more than one miscarriage.

But the causes can be as numerous as they are elusive, and your doctor may only be able to make an educated guess as to why the loss occurred. You can gain an important sense of control, however, by learning about the standard tests that may help identify causes and treatments before you plan your next pregnancy.

Most doctors do not recommend testing after only one miscarriage, since a full series of tests is time-consuming and costly and will probably not yield any significant information about the loss. One miscarriage in a healthy woman who has many childbearing years ahead of her is not treated by doctors as a serious problem, in spite of the emotional impact it might have. Most women require no further treatment after a single miscarriage and 95 percent of them go on to have normal, healthy pregnancies.

Some specialists now recommend that a woman have a complete series of tests after two *consecutive* miscarriages, especially if she is over thirty. With the recent advances in diagnosis and treatment, there is no need for a woman to suffer three miscarriages before beginning the series of tests that might indicate some underlying and treatable difficulty.

Once testing has begun, causes can be clearly identified in under half of all miscarriages. A woman could have hormonal imbalances, complex immunological problems, or uterine malformations that triggered her miscarriage. Or she could have several interrelated causes that may require a combination of treatments.

The fact that doctors are not able to determine a cause in over 50 percent of miscarriages can be enormously frustrating, especially if you have endured weeks or months of testing. When you do not know the cause of your pregnancy loss, you also lack a specific course to follow in trying to prevent a subsequent miscarriage, so that succeeding pregnancies may be fraught with uncertainty and anxiety. You may have to try to become pregnant again with your questions unanswered and your doubts unresolved. If your losses continue, you might have to seek further medical advice to continue your search for guidance and answers.

The following causes of miscarriage are presented, from the most common to the least common. Because miscarriages are the most numerous and complex type of pregnancy loss, a fuller discussion of both causes and treatments is presented in Appendix A.

Genetic and Chromosomal Causes

Half of all miscarriages are triggered by chromosomal and genetic abnormalities. Sometimes a fertilized egg does not develop properly because there is a defect carried in the egg or sperm itself, or the flaw may have occurred spontaneously as the pregnancy began. In either case, the problem is irrevocable from the moment of conception.

Down's Syndrome is the most common chromosomal defect, and the incidence of this disorder increases with maternal age. Other genetic and chromosomal abnormalities are unrelated to the mother's age.

Less research has been done on the effect of paternal age in pregnancy loss, but one study indicated an increased risk in fathers over fifty for defects other than Down's Syndrome. More recent research has centred on the manufacture of sperm, which, unlike the mother's eggs, divide rapidly before fertilization and may be subject to genetic mutations as they grow, especially if the fathers have been exposed to hazardous materials or environmental toxins. Sperm that have been subjected to such mutation can still fertilize an ovum.

Embryos that are too abnormal to grow properly are frequently weeded out by nature in the first trimester. This may be the reason why medical professionals often say that an involuntary loss due to chromosomal or genetic errors 'happened for the best' or that it was 'nature's way.'

If a genetic or chromosomal cause has been determined following a miscarriage, the chances of a similar loss occurring in a subsequent pregnancy vary, depending on the age of the couple and simple probability. Although chromosomal problems in the baby account for a high number of first or random losses (50 percent), only about 6 percent of *recurrent* miscarriages are due to chromosomal causes. Some genetic problems do not originate in the embryo but are passed on by parents and can be determined by a simple blood test. The incidence of recurrence with these types of defects can be quite high.

Hormonal Factors
Immediately following conception, a woman's hormonal system begins a complicated series of secretions to sustain the pregnancy. Once the fertilized egg is firmly established within the uterus, this hormonal interplay is continued by the mother, embryo, and placenta, a complex mechanism that can malfunction and lead to miscarriages. Luteal phase defect, or LPD, is the most common hormonal imbalance associated with early pregnancy loss. In LPD, the menstrual cycle is too short and the endometrial lining of the uterus does not develop properly, rendering it incapable of sustaining a pregnancy.

Some research points to the inability of the hormones of older women to sustain a pregnancy, which may account for the correlation between early losses and maternal age.

Uterine Factors
The uterus, or womb, is the organ that protects and nourishes the pregnancy. If it fails to provide the proper environment, the pregnancy can

miscarry. This can happen when the uterus is malformed either genetically or through uterine growths, illnesses, or exposure to the synthetic oestrogen diethylstilbestrol (DES), although this is a problem rarely encountered in the UK.

It is difficult to associate uterine problems with miscarriage accurately because many women with these defects go on to sustain full-term, successful pregnancies. Some of the more common uterine factors that may cause miscarriage are abnormally shaped uteri, such as a divided uterus or a T-shaped uterus; excessively scarred uteri; and uteri that contain large growths within the muscle wall called fibroids.

Immunological Problems

Immunological disorders in pregnant women generally take one of three forms: (1) antiphospholipid antibody syndrome, in which the mother's immune system turns against her own cells and tissues; (2) lupus, involving a similar attack mounted against the mother's body by her own immune system; and (3) fetal rejection, in which the mother's body attacks the baby as if it were a foreign object. A woman should investigate the possibility of immunological problems if she has had three or more consecutive miscarriages without establishing hormonal, genetic, or other problems.

Infectious Factors

Infections from a variety of organisms may result in early losses by causing serious maternal illness. Recent studies have been unclear as to the correlation between Toxoplasma gondii and Chlamydia, two microorganisms previously thought to cause miscarriage. Many other infectious agents, such as the ones that cause rubella or syphilis, have an effect on pregnancy outcome but have not been implicated in early losses. There is further discussion on the effects maternal health has on pregnancy in Appendix A.

One infectious agent that has been implicated in early loss is T-strain mycoplasma. Very little is known about this microorganism, and diagnosis is difficult, but it can be transmitted sexually and can be harboured in the reproductive tract of either parent.

Antenatal Testing

If chromosomal or genetic problems are implicated in the mother's miscarriage history, or if she is over thirty-five, antenatal testing is encouraged by most doctors. Sadly, the tests themselves may increase the risk of miscarriage. A more complete discussion of the implication of antenatal testing and loss appears in Chapter 8, 'Antenatal Diagnosis and Abortion: The Burden of Choice,' and in Chapter 16, 'Becoming Pregnant Again.'

Injuries or Accidents

A century ago it was generally believed that almost any physical or emotional trauma could cause miscarriages. Since much less was known about pregnancy or miscarriage then, doctors as well as pregnant women would routinely assign the tragedy of their loss to some recent event.

No modern studies have clearly proved or disproved this correlation, but doctors generally feel that if an accident or emotional disturbance didn't harm the mother in any significant way, it would not harm the well-protected baby. This, of course, does not include direct trauma to the mother's abdomen or to the baby, which might occur in a fall or car accident.

The Emotional Aftermath of a Miscarriage

In addition to the sorrow you already feel following your loss, you and your partner may find that the terminology health care professionals use to describe miscarriages adds to your anguish. Like many parents, you may have chosen the word 'miscarriage' to describe your early, unplanned pregnancy loss. However, the correct medical term is 'abortion,' which is generally defined as any pregnancy loss, spontaneous or induced, that occurs in the first twenty-four weeks of gestation.

But the term 'abortion' has been so thoroughly adopted in the media and throughout our society to refer to intentional terminations that parents who hear the word used by health care professionals may feel it implies a deliberate act to end their pregnancy. This term can be upsetting when you are trying to cope with the emotional impact of having lost a baby much against your will.

One woman found the term 'incomplete abortion' distressing, even though she understood the medical definition:

> The phrase was bandied about casualty, the theatre, and the recovery room. I knew intellectually what they meant, that all of the material from the pregnancy had not been spontaneously expelled from my uterus, but it grated on me every time I heard it. It sounded as if I had tried to get rid of my baby and hadn't done a thorough job. It still irks

me. My doctor even used the phrase during my checkup. Medical staff should realize the impact this has and should choose words to use in front of patients that are not so highly charged.

If you have endured several miscarriages, you may also be angry at your doctor for waiting so long before investigating possible causes. Virginia found a new doctor who immediately identified a potential cause following her third miscarriage, which occurred when she was thirty-eight years old:

> My other doctors had the nerve to make me go through three miscarriages before they would start testing. It should be standard after a second consecutive miscarriage, especially for women like me who started so late.

Karen was only in her twenties when she suffered her losses, but she was equally furious when her doctors made her wait until after her third miscarriage before starting tests. 'Even though they didn't find anything particularly wrong,' she explained, 'I felt better knowing we had explored all the avenues before we tried to get pregnant again.'

While sad that a wanted pregnancy has ended, you may be comforted knowing that the pregnancy was probably unhealthy and could not have developed properly. You may agree with the scientists who view early miscarriages as nature's way of dealing with defective embryos. After Annette conceived again following a miscarriage, her husband, Eric, described the feelings he had about her early loss:

> I'm what I guess you'd call a biological realist and believe there was something wrong with that first baby so it couldn't maintain life. It seemed right and proper that the baby we lost should make way for something wonderful and beautiful – these two little healthy girl babies we're expecting now.

You may find, however, that you are not consoled by these explanations and feel they dismiss your need to grieve. You may believe that if everything always happened for the best, you would have had a healthy pregnancy from the beginning. You may long for some acknowledgement of your grief and believe you have reason to be sad that your pregnancy ended.

Julia was upset by the superficial reassurances her husband's family offered after her miscarriage, which only made her realize how little they understood her feelings:

> They did the best they could. But they tried to just pat me on the hand

while they mouthed all the clichés, like 'You can have another baby' or 'It wasn't really a baby yet.' I could not convince them how badly I was feeling.

Medical insensitivity on this issue can make you incredibly angry. Doctors tread a thin line between reassuring you that miscarriages are the most common type of pregnancy loss and recognizing that you feel emotional anguish. If doctors consider miscarriages to be so ordinary, they should understand that grief is an equally unremarkable response. 'I got tired of hearing my doctors dismiss my feelings,' said Vera. 'They kept saying that everyone has miscarriages, as if that were supposed to make my sadness go away.'

Receiving some small recognition of your grief can be comforting, and its absence can make you feel much worse. Susannah recalled how quickly she healed physically after her discharge from the hospital. 'But it was a horrible experience emotionally,' she admitted. 'I was so depressed in the ward, and I was crying. I had just lost a child, and no one acknowledged that.'

In spite of all the emotional trauma you experienced in the first few weeks following your miscarriage, you may feel unexpectedly strengthened by simply surviving the ordeal. 'I know the effect on my life is double-edged,' said Karen in contemplating her five miscarriages. 'I am tremendously sad, but I have also gained compassion and understanding of others because of my losses. Those little babies I never knew still had an impact on my life.'

Experiencing an Ectopic Pregnancy

My husband and I had been trying to get pregnant for a couple of months. My period was a little late and I thought I might be pregnant, but nothing had been confirmed. One night I was on duty at the hospital where I work and I suddenly had a great deal of abdominal pain. At first I thought it was something I had eaten the night before. The pain got worse and I kept getting hotter and hotter. I was going into shock, but didn't realize it. So I went into the bathroom at the hospital and took off my shirt because I was so hot. I was getting dizzy spells, so I lay down on the bathroom floor. Then I started to worry and had this impression that if I didn't stand up and get help, I would die right there on the bathroom floor.

So I used all my efforts to stand up and put on my shirt, but as I opened the door, I fainted into the hallway. This saved my life. Otherwise I would have gone into shock, lost most of my blood supply into my abdomen, and died. But I fainted on a hospital floor, and doctors and nurses came to help. If I had been out shopping, I would never had made it to the hospital alive.

My tubular pregnancy had ruptured right into an ovarian artery. Forty minutes after fainting in the hospital bathroom, I was in surgery. I eventually lost 60 percent of my blood volume from the ovarian artery. This near death became the unfortunate backdrop to my trying to become pregnant again.

TRACY

Ectopic pregnancy, from the Greek root meaning 'displaced,' occurs when a fertilized egg becomes implanted anywhere outside the uterus. Ectopic pregnancies are no longer rare, and the incidence is increasing dramatically. In 1981, one study reported an ectopic pregnancy incidence of 1 in 500 pregnancies in the UK. By 1991, studies were showing rates nearer to 1 in 300 pregnancies.

Close to 98 percent of all ectopic pregnancies occur in the fallopian tubes, but rare cases have been documented in the ovary, in the cervix, or elsewhere in the abdominal cavity. Away from the protective, nourishing environment of the uterus, the growing embryo and placenta cannot survive, although they continue to develop for several weeks. If implantation occurs in a small, contained area, such as a fallopian tube, the greatest danger is that the pregnancy remains undetected and, as it grows, pushes on the sides of the fallopian tube walls until they rupture. Severe internal bleeding is often the result, and it can be fatal.

Women who have experienced one ectopic pregnancy have little more than a 40 percent chance of having a successful pregnancy afterward. This is primarily because of the extensive damage usually done to the fallopian tubes and the increased risk of experiencing a second ectopic pregnancy following any subsequent conception.

Symptoms and Diagnosis of an Ectopic Pregnancy

The symptoms of ectopic pregnancy can be masked as well as varied and may have left you and your partner completely unprepared for the diagnosis. Your doctors may have been equally misled by the symptoms. In fact, misdiagnosis following the first visit to the GP's surgery occurs in roughly 50 percent of all cases of ruptured ectopic pregnancies.

The most common symptom is intense abdominal pain, which might be misdiagnosed if the woman is not aware of an early pregnancy and shows no other signs of being pregnant. The pain usually increases just prior to the rupture of the tube, but then decreases until either infection sets in or the volume of internal bleeding causes severe abdominal pressure.

Some women have described a sudden faintness or weakness, caused by loss of blood following a rupture, even before severe pain is noticeable. About 25 percent of women who suffer a ruptured fallopian tube experience a sharp pain in their neck or one shoulder, due to pressure on nerves from the haemorrhaging blood. Other women experience irregular vaginal bleeding, which might be misinterpreted as a miscarriage if they knew they were pregnant. However, the amount of blood passed in an ectopic pregnancy is usually less than that of a miscarriage. Women who do not realize they are pregnant may think they are having a regular menstrual period.

The earlier an ectopic pregnancy is properly diagnosed, the more likely you will be able to conceive and carry a future pregnancy. If the doctor can treat the ectopic pregnancy before it ruptures, the chances of salvaging damaged tubes and other reproductive organs are greatly increased. Once an ectopic pregnancy is suspected, the doctor can perform several procedures to confirm it.

Abdominal tenderness during a pelvic examination, even if it is not severe, may indicate the internal bleeding associated with an ectopic pregnancy. Blood for a pregnancy hormone blood test should be drawn twice in forty-eight hours to confirm the pregnancy and to see if hormone levels are rising as they should during a normal pregnancy. Other blood tests can rule out the possibility of appendicitis, which has similar symptoms, and scans can provide a picture of the womb and abdomen, often revealing the misplaced pregnancy. However, these tests are not always conclusive. Extensive bleeding can mask the ectopic pregnancy on a scan, and low hormone levels may appear in a healthy pregnancy as well as in a miscarriage or an ectopic pregnancy.

Culdocentesis, a procedure in which a needle is inserted through the vaginal wall into the abdominal cavity behind the uterus, is sometimes performed. If blood is drawn out through the needle, it indicates that internal bleeding, probably from an ectopic pregnancy, is occurring. The doctor can also schedule a laparoscopy, in which a small optical instrument is inserted through an incision in the abdominal wall. The doctor can actually see the fallopian tubes and the ovaries during a laparoscopy, making it one of the most definitive tools in diagnosing an ectopic pregnancy.

Treating an Ectopic Pregnancy

If an ectopic pregnancy is discovered or even strongly suspected, the doctor will move directly into surgery. This is an extreme emergency, and action must be taken immediately to remove the pregnancy, save as much of the reproductive organs as possible, and safeguard the mother's life.

If the pregnancy has developed within the fallopian tube, but the tube has not yet ruptured, it is possible that the pregnancy can be removed and the tube effectively repaired. But once the tube has ruptured, chances are far greater that it must be removed. New microsurgical techniques and laser technology have increased the success of reconstructive surgery following a rupture, but statistics indicate that only about 60 per cent of women conceive at all following an ectopic pregnancy, and of those, 15 percent have yet another ectopic pregnancy.

Although some doctors are currently experimenting with drug therapy to dissolve an ectopic embryo, the primary drug is methotrexate, an agent used in chemotherapy for cancer patients. As a result, most doctors are reluctant to use this method unless an individual case clearly warrants it.

Causes of Ectopic Pregnancy

Fallopian tube problems are the most common factors in the 60 percent of ectopic pregnancies with known causes. This is partially because even healthy fallopian tubes are not straight and smooth, but actually wrinkled on the inside surface, creating little pockets and creases in which a fertilized egg might implant itself and grow.

Infection, however, can make the fallopian tubes flatter and smoother, which may interfere with the fertilized egg's ability to move into the uterus. Hormonal imbalances and reproductive tract malformations, such as very long tubes, have also been implicated in ectopic pregnancies.

In over 40 percent of ectopic pregnancies, a specific cause is never determined, and it is assumed that some other physical problem prevented the fertilized egg from moving through the tube down to the uterus. Unfortunately, no matter what the cause, a woman who has experienced an ectopic pregnancy runs an increased risk of having another ectopic pregnancy following any subsequent conception.

The Emotional Aftermath of an Ectopic Pregnancy

*I*t is upsetting to know that once you have endured one ectopic pregnancy, with each subsequent conception you run the risk of another ectopic pregnancy, surgery, and infertility. But a far graver concern is that another ectopic pregnancy could put your life in jeopardy yet again.

The extensive planning required to contemplate a subsequent pregnancy can be overwhelming and can affect every aspect of your life. You and your partner may avoid work-related trips or holidays to be sure you remain close to medical facilities while trying to conceive. Sacrifices willingly endured for a newborn baby can be unwelcome while merely contemplating a pregnancy.

Tracy had experienced two ectopic pregnancies and felt as if she couldn't plan anything about her life or work for fear of having another. 'Once I realized how vulnerable I was, it spilled into my whole life,' she confessed. 'Just planning the pregnancy was a daunting task.'

Ectopic pregnancies can also leave you and your partner upset and embarrassed by the loss of privacy that occurs when your personal misfortune becomes a medical crisis. Lack of privacy continues to be a problem when you try to conceive again because close medical monitoring is so important. One woman, who was anxious to become pregnant again, described how unsettling it was to have a pregnancy test early in each menstrual cycle. 'I kept thinking I shouldn't have to expose all my hopes and feelings like this once a month,' she admitted. 'I did it because I had to, but it was like watching a pot that never boiled.'

Because ectopic pregnancy is a life-threatening condition, a couple's sexual relationship is often affected. One woman described how the thought of potentially dying as a result of conception was 'very unarousing' to both her and her husband. 'Although we did other things to give each other pleasure and have climaxes,' she recalled, 'we simply were not able to have intercourse for almost a year after my ectopic pregnancy.'

You may find that people who recognize the potential dangers in a subsequent pregnancy can make unusually presumptuous and vexing comments to you and your partner. 'People just didn't want to hear that we were planning another pregnancy,' explained one woman. 'They thought my husband and I were crazy and irresponsible and didn't hesitate to tell us that.'

Vera was equally annoyed when people asked her if she was ready to adopt after her second ectopic pregnancy. 'At the time, my husband and I had different feelings about adoption,' she admitted, 'so we didn't feel like discussing it with outsiders.' While you can't avoid the intrusion of other people's comments, you may feel better if you frankly explain that you need comfort more than opinions or advice.

You may face a special frustration when your grief over losing a pregnancy goes completely unacknowledged. Many people regard an ectopic pregnancy as a medical emergency only and refuse to realize that no matter where your baby was growing, it was still your baby. As Tracy explained:

> I couldn't shake the feeling that the first ectopic was a real baby. She was even a girl to me. She would have been born in June, and every summer I think about how old she would be now.

Your ectopic pregnancy was a real pregnancy that ended in the loss of your baby. Although your feelings of grief may be complicated by serious medical concerns, you still need to mourn your loss, and you deserve support as you recover from your physical and emotional ordeal.

Experiencing a Molar Pregnancy

We had been married for three years when we decided to start a family. When I became pregnant and it appeared to be a normal pregnancy, everything seemed fine. Toward the end of the first trimester, the doctor couldn't find a heartbeat. I should have followed this up with blood tests, which would have indicated the problem. I know I should have, but I have extremely small veins and refused to have the blood tests done. I also felt fine and didn't think anything was wrong.

At that point I changed doctors, and the new one insisted that I go immediately for a scan, and I went that day. I don't remember looking at the ultrasound screen – I have blocked out so many of these painful memories – but I remember being told that there was nothing in the uterus. But they had to have seen the molar pregnancy, even though they didn't say anything to me. I felt so lost.

SONIA

A molar pregnancy – or as it is known medically, a hydatidiform mole – is a pregnancy in which the placenta develops into a mass of fluid-filled sacs that resemble clusters of grapes. There was initially a conception that triggered the formation of the hydatidiform mole, but no baby was ever present in the womb.

A molar pregnancy grows at a regular rate, sometimes even faster than a normal pregnancy, and the uterus expands to accommodate its size. Although this condition is rare, occurring once in every two thousand pregnancies in the UK, it appears to be on the rise.

Women who suffer a molar pregnancy also face an increased risk of developing a rare form of cancer, which although highly treatable is still extremely serious and requires vigilant follow-up medical care.

Symptoms and Diagnosis of a Molar Pregnancy

There are very few physical symptoms of molar pregnancy that can serve as accurate warning signs. Most women experience bleeding and some have nausea and vomiting, but these symptoms can occur in both normal and abnormal pregnancies. Severe nausea accompanying a hydatidiform mole may be caused by high hormone levels resulting from the rapid growth of the placenta. The sudden onset of high blood pressure can also be an indication that a hydatidiform mole has formed. But many women, like Sonia, have no outward symptoms at all. 'It really seemed like a text book pregnancy up until the point when the doctor couldn't find a heartbeat,' she recalled.

A molar pregnancy can be confirmed by a scan, which may indicate the lack of a baby or a heartbeat as well as the particular characteristic appearance of the 'mole'. Occasionally a woman may expel the contents of the womb on her own. A hydatidiform mole tends to produce excessive amounts of the pregnancy hormone HCG at a time when the levels should be falling, or at least levelling off, so a series of blood tests is another important diagnostic tool.

Treating a Molar Pregnancy

Molar pregnancies, like ectopic pregnancies, are among the few pregnancy losses that pose a severe threat to maternal health. Even if the molar pregnancy spontaneously miscarries, it will be necessary to remove remnants of the growth from the uterus, generally by a D&C procedure.

But the real danger comes later. In about 10 percent of molar pregnancies, the woman develops a rare form of cancer from the placental tissue called choriocarcinoma which is nearly always curable with intensive chemotherapy. Doctors generally ask patients who have experienced a molar pregnancy to wait up to two years before conceiving again to make sure the molar pregnancy has not left a cancerous legacy behind. Levels of the pregnancy hormone HCG are measured weekly following a molar pregnancy, because if certain amounts of HCG are still present, the suspicion of malignancy is high.

If you and your partner have experienced a molar pregnancy, you should be assured that this is a rare form of pregnancy loss. As long as you continue to have thorough checkups, you are likely to have other, healthy pregnancies.

Causes of Molar Pregnancy

Although the causes remain obscure, scientists have studied the genetics of molar pregnancy and have uncovered some important clues. A molar pregnancy appears to result from the double fertilization of an 'empty egg,' one in which the nucleus is absent or inactive. Doctors suspect there may be other factors as well, such as genetics and ethnic origin, which may explain the higher incidence of molar pregnancy in Southeast Asia.

A few reports have noted that molar pregnancies occur among sisters, especially if they are twins, and there is a documented risk for women over forty. If a woman has developed one hydatidiform mole, she has a slightly increased risk of having another and should be monitored carefully during subsequent pregnancies.

The Emotional Aftermath of a Molar Pregnancy

Although you and your partner have suffered a molar pregnancy, you still have a very good chance of carrying a healthy baby to term. But succeeding pregnancies are tense and anxiety-ridden. One woman succinctly described her subsequent pregnancy as 'probably the worst time of my life.' Sonia felt she could relax more once she had a healthy baby who was born a year and a half after her molar pregnancy. But even with the pregnancy that produced her second healthy child, Sonia had grave doubts:

> At that point I knew I was capable of having a normal child, but I still worried that the second pregnancy would turn into a molar one, even

after I heard the heartbeat and saw the baby on the scan and knew she was a real baby.

You may also have to confront the reactions of family and friends who are often misinformed about the dangers and risks of molar pregnancies. And because a baby was not actually growing, your need to grieve the loss of the child you had hoped for is often completely overlooked. As Sonia said:

When people are ignorant they don't know what to say. Some people thought I would definitely get cancer and they were fearful of me.

It was hard for me to accept that my conception was a hydatidiform mole, but in my mind the molar pregnancy was still a pregnancy and I grieved that loss.

What Can Help Following Your Early Loss

When you lose a pregnancy in the first trimester, you struggle to gain acknowledgement and validation for the loss of a baby who was real primarily only to you. You may be under the stress of having to seek medical tests or plan for special medical care during your next pregnancy. These additional demands make it especially important for you to recover emotionally from your loss. Whatever type of early loss you have had, if you feel the need to mourn, you should be allowed to do so.

Here are some suggestions that can help you give expression to your grief and deal with the awkward situations unfeeling comments may create:

- Allow yourself time to grieve. This is not a process that can be rushed. Talk about your loss and your feelings with your partner; keep the lines of communication open. Be honest about what the pregnancy meant to you, no matter how brief it was.
- If you feel you need more medical information about your loss, ask your doctor direct questions. If you think you should see a specialist, ask your doctor for a referral or seek a medical consultation with a specialist on your own.
- Don't be surprised if you suddenly feel sad again around the baby's due date or the anniversary of your loss. This 'anniversary reaction' is

an appropriate response, which many bereaved parents experience.

- If you find you are not receiving acknowledgment of your loss from family, friends, and medical staff, seek out other sources of emotional support. Read Chapter 10, 'Finding Solace in Your Religion,' and Chapter 11, 'The Response of Your Family and Friends,' and consider meeting with a psychotherapist or a pregnancy loss support group in your community.

CHAPTER 6

CRISIS PREGNANCIES AND LOSS

W̶hen your loss follows a serious complication during pregnancy, urgent decisions about medical interventions are thrust upon you and your partner, probably leaving you overwhelmed and anxious. You may be worried about your prospects for future healthy pregnancies as well.

The longer your pregnancy lasted, the more time and energy you and your partner committed to maintaining the pregnancy and thinking about the baby. Since some complications can be treated if detected early enough, you may feel additionally upset if the cause of your loss was not identified in time to save the baby.

Doctors are usually quick to intervene in such crisis pregnancies because most result in premature birth. Babies born before thirty-four weeks' gestation have low birth weights and underdeveloped vital organs, which create complications that often lead to newborn death. But treatments for preventing threatened losses and for aiding potentially premature infants are often complex and sometimes experimental, compelling you to make medical and ethical decisions you may feel ill-equipped to handle.

A number of complications in pregnancy can create a medical crisis that may lead to a loss. In a condition called placenta praevia, the placenta grows over the opening of the cervix and can cause haemorrhaging, early delivery, and other serious complications to the mother and the baby.

An equally serious medical emergency can occur if a woman's uterus is weakened from scarring or structural defects, causing the uterus to rupture suddenly as the pregnancy progresses or labour begins. As a result, the mother may haemorrhage and the baby could die. Diabetes and certain infections, such as those caused by the common gastrointestinal bacterium Listeria, may bring on medical crises that can lead to pregnancy loss.

One of the most common crises in pregnancy that can lead to loss is high blood pressure. Some women have a predisposition to this condition before they become pregnant; others may develop high blood pressure after they conceive because of an underlying kidney ailment or other physiological problem exacerbated by the pregnancy. High blood pressure can usually be controlled by bed rest and, occasionally, with medication, but it can become dangerously elevated even with vigilant medical care. High blood pressure is one of the leading causes of maternal death during pregnancy and can trigger early delivery and loss.

The three most common causes of crises in pregnancy related to early delivery and loss are premature labour, premature rupture of the membranes, and cervical incompetence. Although all share certain common issues, each has particular causes, treatments, and emotional consequences that are discussed in this chapter. More detailed information regarding specific treatments is listed in Appendix A.

Issues Common to All Crisis Pregnancies

If your medical crisis progressed to delivery before the thirty-fourth week of your pregnancy, you were forced to confront all the anxieties that accompany the birth of an extremely premature baby. If labour began before twenty-three weeks' gestation, you faced the likelihood of your infant's death shortly after birth. You were probably unprepared for either a very ill infant or your baby's death, even if your condition had been accurately diagnosed and the probable outcome clearly explained to you.

Hopefully, you and your partner had the chance to speak with a neonatologist or fetal medicine specialist who could realistically assess your baby's condition and chances of survival before delivery. Amelia and her husband, Charles, met with two neonatologists while she was in labour during her twenty-third week of pregnancy. The doctors explained that their baby would not be viable if delivered, which allowed Amelia and Charles to decide against intervening in their tiny infant's life should he be born that day. 'Knowing in advance that John wouldn't live long after birth,' acknowledged Amelia, 'helped us say goodbye to him.'

Treatments for premature labour, premature rupture of the membranes, and cervical incompetence often involve bed rest and hospitalizations, which have an enormous impact on all aspects of a patient's life. Extended bed rest and family separations during hospital treatments can take their toll on the most loving relationships. Children at home may especially miss their once active, involved mother tremendously.

Paula underwent treatments for premature rupture of the membranes and found them to be a physical ordeal as well as an emotional one:

> I had my legs up, and my head was lower than my feet. I couldn't eat solid food in case I went into labour at any moment, and I felt I was getting weaker and weaker every day. I couldn't move or go anywhere. I missed my daughter, who wasn't allowed to visit so she couldn't expose me to germs. It was awful, like being trapped while waiting for disaster to strike.

If you and your partner endured an arduous period of trying to maintain a crisis-ridden pregnancy, you may have been surprised when a sense of relief overcame you once the delivery was over, even though it resulted in a loss. If you did not know that relief is a natural response, you may have found it very disturbing.

Relief after the delivery does not mean you didn't want or love your baby, but rather that you welcomed your release from the extreme anxiety, uncertainty, and, for mothers, the physical pain of enduring a crisis pregnancy. Feeling relief does not negate your sense of loss or your need to mourn. Accepting that both relief and sorrow are natural reactions to your loss can help your emotional recovery.

When a crisis pregnancy required bed rest or hospitalization, both parents must adjust to the tragedy of a loss after having endured major disruptions in their family life and work obligations, ultimately in vain. Mothers may be physically weak from their immobilization and should allow themselves ample time to regain their strength. They may find it helpful to build in extra practical and emotional support during this adjustment period, from assistance with housework to psychotherapy, if needed.

You and your partner will also have special medical and emotional needs when you begin to plan a future, possibly high-risk pregnancy. Reading Chapter 14, 'The Impact of Pregnancy Loss on Your Career,' and Chapter 16, 'Becoming Pregnant Again,' can help prepare you for the special challenges involved.

The physical, emotional, and family strains of facing a future high-risk pregnancy may ultimately affect your dreams for the number of children you and your partner plan to have. Marianne, who had lost three children to crisis pregnancies, felt so strongly about the difficulties of maintaining a pregnancy with bed rest, especially once she had a child to care for, that she and her husband decided not to have any more children after their second healthy daughter was born:

I went for a checkup when my youngest was about two years old, and the doctor was talking to us about birth-control methods. He turned to us and said, 'You know, there is no reason why you can't have another baby!' But my husband and I just looked at each other and then at him and said, 'No, two is just great!'

In spite of all the stresses you have endured, you may be struggling to find some purpose to your sorrow that will enable you to mourn and go on with your life. Sometimes this takes the form of an added appreciation for a child born after the loss. 'I think about the fact that we would not have Max if I had been able to keep that other baby,' Paula explained. 'And Max is so special and so wonderful.'

You may also find you are more able to be comforting when friends and family experience sorrow and disappointment. Caroline admitted that her pregnancy loss following a medical crisis enabled her to reach out to others more effectively:

I talk to people who have children with problems or who have experienced pregnancy losses. I feel we are all in it together and that I am more helpful because I truly understand what they are going through. I had good support from family and friends when I went through my loss, and I want to be there for others now.

Experiencing Premature Labour

During my first pregnancy, I was supposed to stop work and rest at home around the twenty-eighth or twenty-ninth week because of my double uterus, but I went into premature labour three weeks before my last scheduled day at work.

I thought something was happening, I felt something, but it was my first pregnancy and I didn't know what to expect. The doctor examined me but couldn't feel anything or see anything, so he thought I was okay. I went on oral ritodrine just in case, but I only had time to take one pill before hard labour began.

My husband was away on a business trip, but I was in too much pain to drive myself to the hospital, so I called one of my best friends to drive me. I lay down in the back seat of her car, and even thought I had never experienced childbirth before, I suddenly felt that the pain had changed, that something more dramatic was happening. We had just pulled into the car park of the hospital when I felt the baby being born. Suddenly it seemed like there were dozens of doctors and nurses and machines all around the back seat of the car.

Olivia was so premature, she only lived a few weeks. We released a balloon from the car park, just like the helium ones we used to bring to her every week to attach to her incubator. AMELIA

As Amelia discovered, premature labour is both a frightening and a frustrating experience. Most parents desperately want their doctor to stop the process, to do anything to save the baby, but unfortunately this is not always possible.

Despite many medical advances in the past three decades, the incidence of premature labour followed by delivery has remained constant, at approximately 10 percent of all live births in the UK. Premature deliveries that are not due to congenital malformations or genetic problems are responsible for almost 75 percent of all neonatal deaths.

Symptoms and Diagnosis of Premature Labour

Premature labour is generally defined as at least six to eight uterine contractions per hour, accompanied by progressive change in the opening or thinning of the cervix between the twentieth and thirty-seventh weeks of pregnancy. But many women find the symptoms of premature labour to be unclear, especially in a first pregnancy, when they are not sure what contractions or other warning signs should feel like. Because early contractions of premature labour are not necessarily painful, some women may not even realize they are in labour.

Even if a woman is not sure what is happening, she may expect her doctor to make a precise diagnosis. But there is so much individual variation in cervical change and uterine contractions that doctors may misdiagnose the condition. This is especially true in the very early stages, when doctors may overtreat contractions that are not necessarily a prelude to labour in order to avoid undertreatment of true labour.

Internal examinations are the best way to see whether the cervix has dilated or effaced. However, doctors usually keep such internals to a minimum because of the risk of introducing infection. Uterine monitors that indicate the strength and frequency of contractions are also employed to help diagnose premature labour. Some doctors prefer to treat most symptoms rather than wait and run the risk of labour progressing so far that it is irreversible.

In spite of the high incidence of premature labour and the opportunity doctors have to observe it, they are usually unable to predict when it will occur. As a result, doctors have focused their efforts on trying to prevent premature labour in women at risk and on trying to stop, or at least slow down, the symptoms once they begin.

Treating Premature Labour

If there is any possibility of stopping premature labour, the doctor will impose bed rest and drinking of fluids at home, hoping that the contractions will slow or stop as soon as pressure is taken off the cervix and the woman is properly hydrated. If this fails, the woman is usually hospitalized for intravenous hydration with saline solution, which can also check or at least curb contractions. If labour stops and the woman is discharged home, her doctor may recommend that she use a small home monitoring device to pick up any recurrence of contractions.

If the contractions do not stop, the next line of defense is treatment with either oral or injected drugs, called tocolytics, to control contractions.

Because all tocolytics have dramatic side effects, including racing heart and low blood pressure, they are used only in clear cases of premature labour and must be carefully regulated. It is a challenge for doctors to balance the efforts to prolong the pregnancy for the baby's safety against the mother's physical stress on powerful drugs. As one doctor expressed it, 'We have to remind ourselves that we are treating a mother here, too.'

Causes of Premature Labour

In most cases, the causes of premature labour are unknown. Sometimes a woman simply begins the process of labour long before the baby is due. As one obstetrician points out, 'As much as we understand labour, no one knows exactly what triggers the strong contractions that help propel the baby into the world.' This makes it hard simply to shut down the triggering mechanism until the baby has been in the uterus long enough to develop sufficient lung power and other critical functions necessary for survival.

Doctors do know that certain wombs cannot expand properly during pregnancy. This may be due to a structural malformation the woman is born with, such as Amelia's double uterus. In other cases, a malformation due to fibroid tumours is acquired as an adult and can fill the space within the uterus so that a normal pregnancy does not have room to grow. A twin pregnancy or excess amounts of amniotic fluid can also occupy more space in the uterus and may trigger premature labour.

Maternal illness such as urinary tract, uterine, and vaginal infections have also been implicated in premature labour. As the bacteria are destroyed in the body, by-products of the process can release potent substances such as prostaglandins, which can cause uterine contractions.

Emotional Aftermath Following Premature Labour

If the cause of premature labour is related to a physical problem, many women are burdened with additional feelings of guilt following a loss. Amelia recalled feeling culpable at the moment of her second premature delivery, knowing that her double uterus contributed to premature labour in each of her pregnancies:

> It crystallized for me when John was born at twenty-three weeks and we knew he wouldn't survive. When I held him I cried and said, 'John, I'm really so sorry.' I guess I held myself responsible. I was aware of my double uterus and knew it figured in these premature births and that part of the problem was intrinsic to me.

But not knowing the cause can be equally painful, rendering you and your partner fearful and anxious about future pregnancies and your hopes for having a family. Stella struggled with the fact that she never discovered the cause of the premature labour that triggered her midterm loss:

> I started to question whether or not I was ever going to have a second child. The sense of futility, of having the loss happen so fast, of going through the high of making it to the second trimester where I thought I would be safe, overwhelmed me. We were back to zero again.

To lose your baby after such a tremendous investment can be extremely difficult. And once you know you are at risk for premature labour, you must take extraordinary precautions the next time you become pregnant. Although this may include weeks or even months of bed rest and hospitalizations, many carefully monitored subsequent pregnancies do result in the birth of healthy babies.

In spite of the profound negative impact premature labour can have, with all of its stresses and sense of loss, you and your partner may find some consequences to be surprisingly positive. After suffering a loss due to premature labour, one woman said of her subsequent high-risk pregnancy:

Our family and friends really came together and worked together to help me manage this last pregnancy. Even with my problems, I would definitely go through another pregnancy again, especially if I believe I can have a baby at the end.

Experiencing Premature Rupture of the Membranes

A couple of days after Paula's amniocentesis, she joined me in Scotland on holiday. She took a nap after her train arrived, but when she awoke and stood up, there was a gush of fluid, and suddenly a pool of blood appeared on the floor. We rushed her to a nearby hospital, but the bleeding stopped by the time we got there. They did a scan, and everything looked fine. The baby had a strong hearbeat.

This gave us an enormous sense of relief, but we decided to cut our holiday short and return home. Once home, Paula had a transvaginal scan and the doctor couldn't see a tear in the sac at all. The doctor felt if Paula kept her feet up and took it easy, everything would be fine. At that point I felt we had been spared and were lucky. We hadn't lost the baby and felt optimistic.

A few days later, Paula woke up in the middle of the night complaining of a warm rush of fluid. We were terrified she was haemorrhaging again and were relieved when we saw it was clear liquid. But she had to keep changing her sanitary pads all day and finally called the doctor, who told her to go to the hospital immediately. A scan showed almost all of the fluid gone, and they assumed Paula would go into labour immediately or would develop a fever from an infection. But she didn't do either, and the fluid reaccumulated.

What followed then were several weeks of hospitalization. The fluid would accumulate and then leak again. The doctor thought the rip in the membranes might heal itself, and we clung to that hope. We were having frequent scans to test the fluid levels and finally, one day, the fluid was all gone. A neonatologist told us that the baby's lungs could not develop properly from that point, that it was over. Paula still hadn't gone into labour, so she had to be induced. It was a harrowing experience.

TED

Like Paula and Ted, you and your partner probably knew that bleeding during pregnancy can be a sign of trouble, but you may not have realized that a loss of clear fluid could be a danger signal as well. Premature rupture of the membranes, or PROM, occurs when the fluid-filled membrane, or amniotic sac, that holds the growing baby breaks before the onset of labour. If the sac tears at term, 80 percent of women will go into normal labour within the next twenty-four hours. But if it occurs before thirty-four weeks' gestation, it can pose severe problems to both the baby and the mother.

The danger to the baby is threefold. Firstly, premature delivery is a major concern, usually occurring within a few days of the onset of PROM. Secondly, once the protective sac has been torn, infection can set in rapidly. Thirdly, once amniotic fluid starts leaking through the tear, adequate volumes of fluid may not be produced quickly enough to serve as a protective buffer for the baby during the remainder of the pregnancy. Risks to the mother include uterine infection and fever, both of which can be managed with antibiotics and delivery of the baby.

Premature rupture of the membranes is responsible for 30 percent of all cases of premature birth in the UK. Usually the cause can never be discovered, but certain infections or specific conditions, such as excess amounts of amniotic fluid, multiple pregnancy, or cervical incompetence, have been implicated in episodes of PROM.

Symptoms and Diagnosis of Premature Rupture of the Membranes

The most pronounced symptom of PROM is a sudden gush of fluid from the vagina followed by persistent, uncontrolled leakage, but other outward signs can be much more subtle. A woman may notice wetness and assume she is having trouble controlling her bladder or experiencing larger amounts of normal vaginal discharge, both of which are common during pregnancy.

Her doctor should confirm the diagnosis by examining samples of the fluid and visually inspecting her cervix. There are several laboratory tests that can help distinguish amniotic fluid from other vaginal secretions or urine. The doctor may also monitor the woman to check for any signs of fetal distress or uterine contractions, or use a scan to determine the amount of amniotic fluid still within the sac. A pelvic examination with a sterile speculum should be done as soon as possible. An examination by hand is usually avoided unless the doctor expects delivery within twenty-four hours, because it increases the chance of infection.

Because of the difficulty in distinguishing between normal vaginal discharge and leakage of amniotic fluid, good communication between the woman and her doctor is especially important in cases of PROM. This can be a problem if she is cared for in a clinic or by a group of doctors in an antenatal GP practice, in which a different doctor examines her at each visit. If this is your situation, you should be aware of the potential for missing a clear diagnosis and insist on thorough testing and as much continuity as possible in any future prenatal care.

Treating Premature Rupture of the Membranes

Once a diagnosis of PROM has been made, the doctor generally recommends complete bed rest in the hospital until delivery. The woman may be placed in the Trendelenburg position, in which her head is lower than her feet, allowing amniotic fluid to pool. Daily monitoring of both the mother and her unborn baby tests for the onset of possible infections. As a pregnancy advances, the amniotic fluid develops its own antibacterial properties, which can help ward off infection. But once an infection has developed in the uterus, it poses a danger to the mother and can cause the death of her baby.

PROM may also cause the umbilical cord to become compressed, which can be fatal for the baby. This can be checked carefully with a fetal heart monitor.

If neither infection nor labour occurs, the doctor may ask the couple whether they want labour induced, to minimize risks to the mother, or if they want to wait to see what develops, in the hopes of increasing the baby's chance of survival. The parents are then forced to balance the risks to the mother's health against the baby's life in the face of great uncertainty.

No matter what the circumstances are, eventually a resolution does come. If scans indicate that too much fluid has leaked and the baby cannot be saved, labour is induced. Labour *must* be induced if laboratory analysis shows that infection has set in or if the mother develops a fever. Although induction or natural labour both provide a clear conclusion to the crisis, labouring for the birth of a baby who cannot survive is both an emotionally and physically painful event.

Causes of Premature Rupture of the Membranes

No one knows what causes premature rupture of the membranes, but several factors have been identified as contributing to the problem.

Infectious agents such as Chlamydia may ascend from the vagina through the cervix to attack and eventually weaken the amniotic sac, while also infecting the fluid and the growing fetus. Group B Streptococcus organisms, which are routinely found in 20 to 25 percent of the vaginal mucus of all pregnant women, can also cause a weakening of the membranes, which could lead to their rupture. Since some of these conditions can be identified and even treated during pregnancy, a thorough medical examination is mandatory following any episode of PROM.

As a baby grows, the stress on the sac increases. If the structure of the sac is defective, its ability to recover from the impact of the baby's growth and movements may be reduced, and it could tear. Genetic and chromosomal abnormalities in the baby can also trigger premature rupture of the membranes.

Sometimes a combination of conditions could be responsible for PROM. Most women never discover what caused their fluid to leak, and are left anxious and uncertain about what will happen in a subsequent pregnancy.

Emotional Aftermath Following Premature Rupture of the Membranes

If episodes of premature rupture of the membranes plagued your pregnancy through weeks of hospitalization, the attempts to save the baby probably whipped you and your partner back and forth from despair to hope almost daily. If labour was eventually induced, you may have felt a sense of relief when there were clear medical reasons for ending your ordeal. Paula and Ted were forced to accept that their baby was no longer viable after spending weeks trying to save their pregnancy. 'It was like a great sense of relief washed over us,' Ted recalled. 'We were grateful it wasn't a marginal situation anymore, that it was now clear-cut. The decision was finally taken out of our hands.'

Once you have suffered from premature rupture of the membranes, you must face the chance of encountering episodes in future pregnancies. Since you will have a 21 percent chance of experiencing PROM again in each subsequent pregnancy, you must be prepared for the possibility of extensive hospitalizations and difficult choices following each conception.

Losing a baby following premature rupture of the membranes may cause you to search for some consolation that will give you hope and rekindle your desire for another baby. Your priorities may shift to accommodate new goals. Bert felt that his twenty-six-week loss related to PROM and other factors put much of his life into perspective. 'The most important thing to me was my wife, that she was okay,' he admitted. 'And we realized how much we truly want to have a child and only hope that it will be possible.'

Experiencing Cervical Incompetence

I had lost babies at seven weeks, twenty weeks, and twenty-seven and a half weeks. There were a combination of factors in the losses, but after the third loss, of our son who lived just a few minutes, my doctor and I decided to send me to a nearby teaching hospital. They felt that one of my problems was an incompetent cervix and told me that I would have to have a stitch put in my cervix to keep it closed once I was pregnant again.

I had the stitch put in at fourteen weeks in my next pregnancy. I went home and saw the doctor about a week later. The stitch had torn loose and ripped my cervix. At this point, it started to get to me. It seemed that up until our pregnancy losses everything else in our lives had fallen into place. This seemed so frustrating and unfair.

After they fixed the stitch, I stayed in the hospital five months. My legs were up and my head was lower, so as the pregnancy advanced I started to do less and less. I played a mental game with myself. There was so much time ahead of me. After so many losses, I tried to think how lucky and temporary my current situation was. It all seemed worth it when our healthy daughter was born at thirty-eight and a half weeks.

MARIANNE

The cervix is a narrow, ring-shaped structure at the base of the uterus that opens into the vagina. The cervix consists mostly of non-muscle fibre called collagen, and opens during labour in increasing amounts that are measured in centimetres of 'dilation.' During this time it also goes through a process of becoming shorter and thinner, called 'effacement.' However, in a diagnosis of cervical incompetence this ring of fibre begins thinning and opening long before the pregnancy reaches full term, usually without contractions.

This condition generally appears during the second trimester of pregnancy and is surprisingly difficult to diagnose accurately. It is also difficult to determine how many women are afflicted with cervical incompetence, since calculations vary widely. One estimate states that up to 20 percent of all losses in the midtrimester of pregnancy are related to cervical incompetence. Another states that true cervical incompetence is quite a rare phenomenon and tends to be over diagnosed.

Symptoms and Diagnosis of Cervical Incompetence

The symptoms of cervical incompetence fall into two categories: those that a woman can feel or see, and those that are observed by her doctor. It is important that both sets of symptoms be monitored constantly, beginning with the second trimester of any pregnancy at risk for this condition.

Symptoms that a patient can see or feel include vaginal bleeding, or increased vaginal discharge, especially if it is mucousy. A woman may also feel pressure in her pelvis or experience pain similar to cramping. A classic case of incompetent cervix will *not* be accompanied by the strong uterine contractions associated with labour.

Signs that the doctor checks through an internal examination all involve determining the condition of the cervix, such as effacement and dilation, especially if these signs are not accompanied by uterine contractions.

If a woman has had one or more second-trimester losses of undetermined causes, but without labour having to be induced, her doctor should regularly check the condition of her cervix during any subsequent pregnancy by looking at it with the aid of a speculum and performing internal examinations. If the cervix is slightly effaced or opened, or if any of the membranes seem to be showing through the cervical opening, cervical incompetence should be suspected. Scans can be used to measure the length of the cervix, but it is not always conclusive.

Since there are no straightforward criteria for diagnosing cervical incompetence, it is important that the doctor have an understanding of the patient's complete medical history, especially if she has had more than one second-trimester loss suspected to be from cervical incompetence. This history is crucial because if she has had multiple births, pregnancy losses, or D&C's, she may not maintain a tightly closed cervix during subsequent pregnancies and may still experience full-term deliveries.

Probable Treatment for Cervical Incompetence

The primary treatment for cervical incompetence is a cervical cerclage, or stitch. If a woman has a history of cervical incompetence, or if she is showing clear-cut symptoms of cervical incompetence, the cerclage can be placed in and around the cervix, pulling it into a tightly closed position. This procedure requires some form of anaesthesia and a brief hospitalization, usually at the end of the first trimester. There are more risks if the cervical cerclage is placed after eighteen weeks' gestation or once the cervix has opened two to three centimetres. No cerclage is attempted if the cervix has opened four centimetres or more. The cerclage is usually removed in the thirty-seventh week of pregnancy, before labour begins, so it will not tear the cervix as it begins to open.

Success rates for cerclages are difficult to calculate, but some doctors report that using the cervical cerclage prior to dilation on women who have experienced previous cervical incompetence enables 80 percent of them to have full-term pregnancies. Complications of the cerclage include bleeding, leaking of amniotic fluid through ruptured membranes, infection to either the mother or the unborn baby, and the onset of labour.

If cervical incompetence is not detected until the cervix has dilated, or if the patient had a cerclage and developed complications in spite of the stitch, bed rest is recommended. Complete bed rest is generally best achieved in the hospital, where the woman can be cared for by professional staff twenty-four hours a day.

Uterine abnormalities that are related to cervical incompetence pose a more difficult problem. Some, such as a uterus divided by a wall of tissue, or septum, can be surgically corrected if necessary; others cannot routinely be corrected through surgery. And surgery has its own risks, such as scarring, which could create additional problems in a subsequent pregnancy.

Possible Causes of Cervical Incompetence

It used to be that poorly done D&C procedures associated with illegal abortions were the primary cause of cervical incompetence, but since the legalization of abortion, these statistics have dropped dramatically. Most cervical incompetence is now traced to uterine or cervical abnormalities a woman is born with, especially a cervix that is unusually short.

Some spontaneous cases of cervical incompetence show up in women with no known risk, generally after one or more full-term pregnancies. These cases may have resulted from an undetected tear in the cervix or other cervical damage that occurred during the delivery of a previous child. Cone biopsy, a form of cervical surgery, was once implicated in cervical incompetence, but more recent studies have disputed this correlation.

Emotional Aftermath Following a Loss Due to Cervical Incompetence

Even the medical term 'incompetent cervix' may give a parent pause. Some believe it implies a degree of ineptness on the part of the mother, who should not be made to feel guilty about a structural cervical problem she did not cause. Ruth strongly objected to this language:

> It was a horrible terminology to me because it made me feel as if the medical profession was saying that I wasn't quite good enough to be a mother. My cervix was short, and I could visualize that. A short cervix that I couldn't control didn't seem as judgmental to me as an 'incompetent' cervix.

If you and your partner experienced a pregnancy loss through cervical incompetence, you should expect to have special medical precautions taken during each subsequent pregnancy. The recurrence of cervical incompetence is relatively high, so future pregnancies are anxious pregnancies; the innocent expectation of a textbook pregnancy can no longer be yours.

The increase in the number of doctor's appointments can be a drain on your time and energy, adding to your tension about the pregnancy. Laura, who had lost one baby because of cervical incompetence, described what this medical vigilance was like:

> In my next pregnancy, I saw my doctor weekly from twenty weeks onwards, at my request. From thirty-two weeks on I was attached to a fetal monitor weekly, and at thirty-five weeks I also started having a scan every week. All this made me extremely anxious.

You and your partner may be yearning for a way of accepting your sorrow, of integrating it into your life so you can believe your prematurely born infant had not lived, however briefly, in vain. Amelia felt she had established a strong connection with her baby through weeks of hospitalization, even though his premature birth could not be stopped and he lived only about two hours:

> John became a source of companionship for me while I was hospitalized. I actually talked to him and felt we were allies fighting the battle together. Other people came to visit me when it was convenient for them, but John was always there. John was incredibly loyal.

Marianne, who suffered from cervical incompetence, ultimately felt her losses had a bittersweet meaning:

> My losses helped me; they taught me to learn what was important in life and what wasn't. People who experience tragedy are more sensitive to others. Not that I would wish sorrow on anyone, but if it happens, we might as well try to make it a part of our lives and not deny it. And we should try to grow from it.

What Can Help Following Your Loss Due to a Crisis Pregnancy

A loss following a crisis-ridden pregnancy poses particular problems. You and your partner had already invested a great deal of time and energy in the pregnancy, perhaps after days or weeks of hospitalizations or home bed rest. Such sacrifices probably added to your bitter disappointment and frustration when your pregnancy ended in a loss, compounding your feelings of grief.

Here are some suggestions to help you cope with your loss:

- You may feel guilty if you experience a sense of relief when a difficult pregnancy has ended. Relief is a common reaction to the uncommon stress you have endured and doesn't mean you were uncaring toward your baby.
- You may also be extremely angry about your loss, especially if you endured bed rest or other stressful medical interventions. Now that you know you have an underlying medical problem, try to channel your energy into finding the best medical care during your next pregnancy.
- Try not to berate yourself for making decisions about medical care that seemed to pit the mother's interests against your baby's. Balancing these issues is extremely difficult, especially when the outcome is uncertain.
- If your crisis pregnancy required bed rest or hospitalization, take into account your need for time to regain your physical strength and to re-establish your relationship with your partner, as well as time to grieve once you are back home.

•••••••••••••

CHAPTER 7

STILLBIRTH AND NEWBORN DEATH

*I*f your baby was stillborn or died shortly after delivery, you experienced childbirth, but it was a tragic event instead of the happy moment you had anticipated. You were committed to the pregnancy, nurtured it, and planned for the birth of your child. Instead, you now face an unfathomable grief.

Losses beyond the first trimester are less common than early miscarriages. Fourteen percent of all pregnancy losses occur in the second trimester and 6 percent in the third. Yet the causes of both stillbirth and newborn death are numerous. Problems with the structure, positioning, or functioning of the placenta or umbilical cord; maternal illness; premature delivery for any reason; birth defects in the baby; and low birth weight have all been implicated in precipitating later losses. While the cause of many newborn deaths can be determined, over 50 percent of all stillbirths remain unexplained.

After experiencing a loss so late in your pregnancy, you may move through intense and open grief reactions, especially if you saw your baby and said goodbye. If you have no other children, the shock of such a sad outcome to your pregnancy confronts you with an identity confusion in which you may wonder, 'Am I really a parent?' You can be left with the painful contradiction of feeling like a childless parent.

Issues Common to All Stillbirths and Newborn Deaths

*L*ike many parents, you may begin to feel guilty, assuming that you somehow caused or might have prevented this tragedy. If your loss was triggered by environmental or genetic causes, your sense of responsibility for being exposed to dangerous toxins or passing on a defective gene may compound your grief. Even if you know the tragedy was beyond your control, you may still succumb to guilt, since blaming yourself is one way of trying to rationalize an incomprehensible loss.

Although Wendy realized that her baby daughter died from a congenital heart defect she could not possibly have caused, she still felt guilty. 'I always wanted a girl,' she explained, 'and in a way I worried that was why she had died – because I preferred to have a girl and was being punished for wanting one sex more than the other.'

You may find yourself wishing that you had received different antenatal care, believing you could have avoided your tragedy had you been more vigilant. Even when your doctors have assured you there was no way to prevent your loss, you can still be haunted by a longing to have done more.

Roger, whose first child was stillborn after the placenta stopped functioning properly, continued to wonder if the problem might have been detected if his wife had been classified as a high-risk mother and under more constant medical care. 'There was little solace for us in knowing we hadn't caused the loss,' he admitted.

If your pregnancy was complicated by medical problems that required bed rest or surgery for the mother, your loss can seem excruciatingly unjust. 'My sense of unfairness was heightened by having been bedridden for so long both times,' admitted Amelia after she lost a second premature baby. 'It seemed as if my husband and I had suffered enough just trying to hold on to the pregnancies.'

Late losses can also occur with no warning signs. The mother may have experienced a problem-free pregnancy, which gave her, her partner, and her doctor a sense that all would continue to go well. If she was under thirty-five, with no family history of abnormal births, her doctor may have considered her too young to be given antenatal tests that could have revealed a problem. Parents' shock and grief at losing a baby who had seemed fine for so many months can be overpowering.

Once you accept that neither you nor your medical care caused your loss, you can still feel intense frustration over not having been able to protect your baby from harm. However blameless, you may feel you failed your infant, who was vulnerable and dependent. These feelings may intensify when you return home to face the baby's room, complete with cot and layette. You and your partner may have even moved to a bigger place or bought your first house, which is rendered large and empty by your loss.

It is important to analyse and trust your feelings before deciding what to do with the baby's room and layette. Don't rush into a decision that doesn't feel right to you because family or friends are pressuring you, or because you think it's the proper thing to do. Some bereaved parents want the baby things packed up and out of sight before the mother returns from the hospital, so the house doesn't feel like a baby is still expected. Others find the layette a poignant reminder of their love, and they spend quiet moments in the baby's room remembering and grieving, and eventually hoping and planning for another baby.

While she was pregnant, Irene had gathered a few baby things in her flat because she wanted the first days after the birth to be a special, quiet time for her new family. Her baby was due in August, and she didn't want her husband to have to run around shopping in the summer heat. Irene discovered that after her daughter was stillborn, it gave her courage to see the baby things and that their presence helped confirm her commitment to have another child. 'I had made the cot bumpers and sheets myself,' she explained, 'and when I put them away I said to myself, "I *will* use these someday."'

Having this tangible connection to your baby can provide an appropriate expression of love and grief in the early stages of mourning, enabling you, your friends, and your family to achieve another level of acceptance. This happened for Amelia and Charles, who had prepared a room for their premature daughter, who died unexpectedly after being cleared to go home. They discovered that entering their baby's room and being able to see and touch Olivia's pictures, toys, and clothing gave concreteness to her existence, their love for her, and, ultimately, their need to say goodbye.

This crystallized for Amelia one afternoon when a friend brought her three-year-old daughter Sarah for a visit:

> We were upstairs and Sarah said, 'Is that Olivia's room? Can I see it?' We went through Olivia's photo album, too, which was in the room. Sarah's only experience with death had been Olivia's dying, and I wondered if this was going to be okay for her. When we got to the end of the photo album, Sarah didn't seem afraid at all. Actually, going into Olivia's room and looking at the album put all the questions to rest that Sarah had been asking about death, and it helped us enormously, too.

You may find yourself in the awkward position of having to cancel arrangements for child care or other household help that were made in anticipation of a normal birth. Molly had hired a lady to start cleaning on a weekly basis after her baby was due. When her son was stillborn, Molly was so distraught she alternately kept putting off and forgetting to call the cleaning lady to tell her the news. The cleaning lady finally called her. 'Before I could say anything, she wanted to know if I had the baby yet and was it a boy or a girl,' remembered Molly. 'All I could do was say the baby died and hang up on her.'

Most parents prefer to have a friend or family member call to explain the loss and the change in plans, but again, trust your own inclinations. No matter who makes the call to cancel arrangements, it is best to do it promptly, to avoid the pain and embarrassment of having the cleaner or childminder call first for news of the baby.

Once parents have managed to absorb their loss and deal with issues and decisions they can control, mothers must still struggle with their body's response to the pregnancy, which is both a physical and emotional reminder of the loss. Even if a woman had injections to prevent lactation, her milk may come in, reminding her how disastrously amiss it is to have her breasts so full of milk with no baby to nurse.

All of these sensations and dilemmas conspire to make you and your partner feel the loss of your roles as parents as well as the loss of your child. Lucy, whose newborn lived only a few hours, found this loss of motherhood especially troubling:

When Mother's Day came around the following month, I just felt awful. Technically I wasn't a mother anymore. It seemed to me that caring for a child was what makes us parents and that not being able to continue caring for a child took that away.

Another mother, however, felt strongly that her stillborn daughter had enabled her and her husband truly to become parents:

I think Mary made us parents, because even though we didn't have a baby in the house, we still loved this child. And that's the sadness of pregnancy loss. You have the love for your child that does indeed make you parents; only you don't have the child.

Experiencing a stillbirth or newborn death makes subsequent pregnancies extremely trying, since no point in the pregnancy ever seems safe, even if your chances of delivering a healthy baby are good. 'I was convinced my next baby would die the same way,' said Molly of the healthy pregnancy that followed her stillbirth, 'but I also knew nobody wanted to hear about that, so I had the added burden of keeping the fear inside.'

Once your loss is behind you, you must grapple with your sorrow and try to integrate this tragedy into your life. You will never forget the death of your baby, but you can find new richness in your life once you have absorbed your loss and learned to go on. Gail and her husband had lost three babies to a rare combination of genetic factors, and struggled with the impact that losing the babies had on their lives:

> What I found especially upsetting about the losses was that I was raised to feel if you work hard enough you will get whatever you wanted. 'It's up to you' was a phrase we heard a lot around our house when I was a kid. But it's not, and pregnancy loss teaches you that. Yet we didn't want to use our bad luck as a crutch to become unhappy. We both wanted to go on with life, to try to have other children. And we did.

Irene and her husband were able to discover a positive legacy amid their sorrow following their daughter's stillbirth:

> After Mary was stillborn, I became more sensitive to other people's feelings. I might even go overboard now. I try to help people and be more sensitive to other people's grief and sorrow. I think it affected my husband, too, in the same way, in being more sensitive. This is our daughter's gift to us.

Experiencing a Stillbirth

I was so excited about the pregnancy. It was our first, and it had gone so well. I worked right up to the eighth month. One night in the ninth month, my husband, Roger, and I were eating in a restaurant and I felt some violent movements in my womb. Three days later, the baby didn't move at all. I went to the GP, but she couldn't find a heartbeat. By the next day I had started labour on my own and was admitted to the hospital, where our baby was born dead.

SALLY

Sarah and Roger had experienced a stillbirth, a tragedy that befalls over four thousand couples each year in the UK alone. Stillbirth is a contradiction of what we are led to expect in life: death comes before birth, stillness replaces movement, birth becomes an ending instead of a beginning.

Because of this disparity, the symptoms of grief can be exceptionally strong following a stillbirth. Some parents experience aching arms and hear phantom crying for days or even weeks after learning of their baby's death. It is hard to accept that something has gone so drastically wrong after long months of anticipation. Parents can feel cheated when their child is stillborn, after investing so much time in the pregnancy and enduring childbirth – all for nothing.

Diagnosing and Treating a Stillbirth

Symptoms of stillbirth are sometimes difficult to perceive. Even the most active baby can be still for long periods of time in its mother's womb. In the last stages of development before birth, babies rest and often enter a state of deep sleep that can last forty to sixty minutes. Once the baby has grown considerably in the final month of pregnancy and the head is engaged into the pelvis, it cannot move as freely in the womb as it once did. The occasional kick and shift of position is about the most movement a full-term baby can manage in the final two to three weeks before birth – and these are often the abrupt movements more closely associated with the baby's sleep state. Many healthy but subtle fetal movements, such as thumb-sucking, are not even perceptible to the mother. Some women, such as Sarah, experience violent movements prior to a stillbirth, after which the baby becomes uncommonly still. Others may perceive the stillness only after one or two days have passed.

The most immediate means of diagnosing a stillbirth is to listen for the baby's heartbeat. Since fetal heartbeats cannot always be heard through stethoscopes, doctors often use a hand-held device called a sonicoid. If this is inconclusive, a full scan is scheduled. Both fetal movement and a baby's heartbeat can be seen immediately by full ultrasound scan, and in their absence, a diagnosis of stillbirth is accurately confirmed almost 100 percent of the time.

Until relatively recently, there was little doctors could do to hasten the birth of a baby who had died *in utero*, and the woman was forced to carry the baby until the onset of natural labour. Waiting for labour poses little medical danger to the mother, unless it is dealyed for a month or more after the death. But the psychological impact of carrying a dead baby while looking very pregnant is difficult to handle, especially if labour does not begin for days, or even weeks, following the diagnosis.

Although waiting for the onset of natural labour may be the safest medical course to take, many doctors are willing to induce labour to spare parents the agonizing delay before a futile, spontaneous delivery. These induction methods have been in practice for over a decade and include prostaglandin vaginal suppositories or Syntocinon drip. But even with induction, labour can be full, long, and difficult.

Causes of Stillbirth

There are approximately 3,700 stillbirths in the UK each year. In approximately 50 percent of cases, no specific cause can be determined. Of the remaining half, the primary reasons fall into three basic categories: problems with the structure or functioning of the placenta or umbilical cord; maternal illnesses or conditions that affect the pregnancy; and birth defects in the baby, caused by chromosomal or genetic abnormalities.

One of the most common causes of stillbirth is the premature separation of the placenta from the uterine wall, which is called placental abruption. Normally the placenta does not begin separating from the uterus until after birth has occurred, but if this process begins before or during labour, the baby's lifeline for oxygen and nutrients is cut off at the source – the mother's body. Women who have one early placental separation leading to stillbirth have a 10 percent chance of experiencing a second abruption. If a woman has had two abruptions, her chances of experiencing another in a subsequent pregnancy are greater than 25 percent.

If a pregnancy goes longer than it should, the placenta can stop functioning properly. Structural defects in the placenta and the umbilical cord can also cause stillbirth. Sometimes a kink or knot forms in the cord, cutting down on the flow of blood and oxygen to the baby. A cord can become wrapped around the baby's neck or some other part of its body either before or during birth with the same effect, one that is often accelerated during the stress and pressures of labour. If the cord prolapses, or comes out of the uterus prior to delivery, it can be squeezed, cutting off the baby's blood supply.

Many maternal illnesses can cause stillbirth, primarily because the mother's health affects the functioning and well-being of the placenta. Since the placenta absorbs diseases and drugs from the mother's body, it can be so adversely affected that adequate nutrients and oxygen do not cross over to the baby. Lupus, hypertension, diabetes, pre-eclampsia, and infections such as syphilis, listeria, and rubella have all been implicated in stillbirths. Smoking cigarettes can inhibit the flow of oxygen through the placenta, and the use of cocaine can cause the placenta to constrict, inhibiting the transport of nutrients to the baby and leading to stillbirth.

Many illnesses implicated in stillbirth can be treated during a subsequent pregnancy, but the sad fact remains that stillbirths often occur to women with no known high-risk factors.

Chromosomal defects account for 15 to 20 percent of all stillbirths. Down's Syndrome babies, for example, have more than a 30 percent chance of being stillborn. Malformations that are not chromosomal in nature, such as urinary tract obstructions and gastrointestinal tract malformations, can also cause stillbirth. A baby born with multiple congenital anomalies will not necessarily be harmed by the individual defects, but might not be able to sustain life inside the womb because of the combined impact of the abnormalities.

Stillbirth can occasionally occur as a result of an abnormal labour and delivery. The placenta may pull away from the uterine wall during labour, or the umbilical cord might become constricted during delivery. Fetal monitoring is generally so routine in hospitals during labour that such crises can usually be determined, and interventions, such as caesarean deliveries, implemented to prevent the baby's death. However, a woman may arrive at the hospital too late for her baby to be saved if her labour was quick and the damage has already occurred. In the case of a baby with severe congenital defects, it is also possible that the infant could not survive the stress of labour and delivery.

Once you have experienced a stillbirth, it is very important to try to determine a cause, especially if you are planning future pregnancies. An autopsy can help determine the cause of death, or at least rule out some possible reasons for the stillbirth. A biopsy and genetic testing, or karyotyping, of your baby's tissues should be done immediately after delivery. Even if another, more obvious cause seems readily apparent, such as the cord being wrapped around the baby's neck, these tests assure that all underlying causes have been considered. The baby might have had Down's Syndrome or a genetic defect that could have precipitated its death *in utero*, a risk you may want to examine before planning subsequent pregnancies.

If the baby was normal in every way but your pregnancy suffered for some random and unpredictable event, such as a cord accident, your chances of having another healthy pregnancy are very good. A subsequent pregnancy would not necessarily be considered high-risk, and your doctor might recommend routine medical care. Tests that evaluate the baby's health while still in the womb, such as kick charts and scans, can be reassuring options you may want to discuss with your doctor.

Emotional Aftermath Following a Stillbirth

L ike many parents who experience stillbirth, you may have been upset by having to wait for labour to begin naturally. 'I knew Sarah's doctor felt it was best for our having future children that labour not be induced,' explained Roger when he learned his first child would be stillborn, 'but it seemed so horrible for Sarah to have to carry the baby around and wait.'

In some ways, however, waiting may have helped you deal with the loss more effectively. You had time to absorb the tragic news and think about decisions you and your partner would face after delivery, such as holding and naming your baby or having an autopsy and planning a burial. The time delay may also have allowed you to feel somewhat more emotionally prepared for your difficult delivery.

Gloria and her husband preferred to wait for labour to begin once they learned their unborn baby had died, and were pleased to find the hospital staff supported their wishes. 'We asked if we could go home until I went into labour spontaneously,' she remembered, 'and my doctor agreed. We wanted the birth to be as natural as possible, as we had originally planned, with as much privacy as possible.'

If you chose to wait, you probably preferred to stay indoors to avoid dealing with people's comments about your pregnancy. 'I thought if one more bus driver cheerfully asked me when my baby was due,' recalled one mother as she waited for labour with her stillborn child to begin, 'I would start screaming and not be able to stop.'

Once you delivered your stillborn baby, you may have been able to marvel at the baby's beauty and innocence, no matter what the cause of the stillbirth. Roger remembered how difficult this seemed at first:

> The hardest thing was to hold him in my arms, but I'm glad I did. He had all his little toes. He was a very normal-looking baby. I just rocked him and cried uncontrollably as I looked at his round face and nose – his little ski nose – and his little lips. It was so important to hold him.

Even with the finality of the stillbirth, you may have felt as if your nightmare were just beginning. 'Leaving the hospital without the baby was the toughest,' admitted Roger in recalling the day after his stillborn son's birth. 'It seemed so very wrong.' Each event related to the stillbirth weighs heavily in your thoughts, and you may find yourself reliving the labour and birth of your baby over and over again.

As you gradually absorb your sorrow and loss, you may also become more aware of the profound effect your stillborn child has had on your life. 'Jason brought my wife and me closer together,' Roger remembered. 'It is one of his legacies to us.'

Molly had turned to friends and relatives for comfort after losing her stillborn son. When she found that many people couldn't handle her and her husband's pain, it seemed to magnify their loss, and she vowed to help others through this difficult time. She trained to be a befriender with SANDS the pregnancy loss support group that had helped her cope with her stillbirth. Although the work is emotionally demanding, Molly finds that it helps confirm the positive effect her son's brief existence has had on their lives:

> I feel passionately about trying to help others. I try very hard now to reach out to people in the same way that I found helpful. This not only helps them, it is another way of establishing Nathaniel's existence for me. Nathaniel *was* real. He was our son.

Experiencing a Newborn Death

Ashley was born and died on New Year's Day. I went into labour on schedule and was given Syntocinon, so it progressed quickly. When Ashley was born, the delivery room got very quiet. The doctors rushed her out of the room and said nothing to us. I was taken to recovery, and all the doctor told my husband, Peter, was that he had to be strong.

Later we learned that our baby was born with severe congenital anomalies. She lived fifty minutes. Peter told me when she died. He brought her in for me to see, wrapped in a pink blanket. That is when it hit me. Peter wouldn't be a father. We wouldn't be taking Ashley home.

SYLVIA

Every year about 800,000 babies are born in the UK and 500 of those live less than a month. As the parent of one of those babies, you desperately need your partner's support at a time when neither of you is in the condition to provide it. It is very hard to accept that a newborn does not have a good chance of survival and you must endure the torment of uncertainty about your baby's future as you watch your child struggle for life in the hospital.

If your baby was premature, you may have had some time to absorb the shock and sorrow of your child's condition before death occurred. But no matter when you realized your newborn was seriously ill, the joy that normally surrounds the birth of a baby is transformed into doubts and fears for your child's well-being.

You may have been confused and overwhelmed by the medical choices regarding your baby's care that were suddenly thrust on you. Even if the baby's prognosis was bleak, avoiding medical intervention may have seemed tantamount to abandoning the child you had nurtured and loved during the pregnancy. Lucy responded to her newborn son's multiple defects by requesting that everything possible be done for him:

> I remember telling the doctors, 'Save him! Save him!' but there were no choices really. His genetic problems were so severe. There were no decisions to make, so we didn't have to face any. Christopher lived only four hours.

On the other hand, facing major decisions about surgery, removal of life support systems, and other interventions in an infant's care can cause additional anguish to already over-burdened parents. Adam and Lisa's baby daughter was not expected to live because of severe congenital anomalies and was placed in the neonatal intensive care unit until she died. Even knowing that her life would be brief, the couple was not spared a series of medical decisions that eventually created friction between them. Since the baby could not suck on her own, the doctors asked the distraught parents if they wished to have a feeding tube inserted through her nose. 'I didn't agree with the feeding and the use of the tube,' acknowledged Adam. 'I didn't see the need for prolonging her misery and our agony. We knew death was just a few hours away.'

Lisa felt differently and asked the doctors to insert the tube:

> I couldn't bear the thought that on top of everything else she was suffering, that she would also be hungry. But when they tried to insert the tube, Lara winced and cringed and they felt they were hurting her more than helping her, so they left it out. I still have a problem with the whole issue and the antagonism it created between us.

Sorting through conflicting medical information from experts can be extremely perplexing. Amelia and Charles's premature daughter had been on a ventilator from birth, and her short life was a roller coaster of hope and fear for her parents, emotions that often alternated in frequent succession. One day, after their daughter had been transferred to a more sophisticated neonatal intensive care unit in a different hospital, the doctor who headed the unit asked to have a meeting with Amelia. The new doctor suggested that their baby should continue on the ventilator and stay on it for as long as two years:

> I was caught by surprise, since there had been no previous conversation about this topic. In fact, at the hospital where our daughter was born, no goal was more important than getting babies *off* the ventilator, because eventually it causes its own damage. After two years on a ventilator, our baby probably would not have been able to move well, swallow, cry, or even eat normally.

Caught off guard and feeling especially vulnerable because her husband wasn't available at that moment, Amelia found the choices surrounding her infant's care and survival were suddenly clarified, and she responded from her heart. 'I looked at all the doctors present at the meeting and said, "I am speaking for both my husband and myself most emphatically, that we will *never* choose that kind of life for our child,"' she recalled.

Experiences like Amelia's may have left you concerned about how much authority you ultimately had regarding medical interventions in your baby's care. You may have wondered what your legal rights were and worried that a doctor could decide on medical treatment for your child without honouring your wishes or asking your permission. The notion of strangers making such fundamental decisions about your baby and your family's life may have been frightening. Hopefully you had access to a second expert medical opinion when faced with these difficult circumstances.

If your baby had been very ill, she may have been attached to monitors and other medical apparatus, or have been placed in an incubator. She may have looked exceptionally fragile and made you afraid that touching her might jostle delicate medical instruments and cause harm. You might deeply regret not having been able to hold and cuddle your ill newborn because of intimidating medical equipment. Once your infant died, and the tubing and monitors were removed, you may have found it comforting to cradle your baby in your arms as you had longed to do while the baby was alive.

Amelia recalled one of the nurses recommending a touching ritual immediately after her premature baby died:

> It seemed so bizarre at first, but so right after we did it. She suggested that we give Olivia a bath. It was wonderful! It was the first time Olivia wasn't encumbered with any electrodes and tubes to handle.

She was still warm and pink; it was as if she wasn't dead. We put her in one of her little outfits. We stayed a little longer and left and went home. The last thing we saw of Olivia that day was her dressed in the little pink and white stretchy suit we had put her in. It was a wonderful memory.

But even if you saw and held your infant, you may have also grappled with the distress of having so little time with your baby. You may have wondered if your tiny child could really know how much you loved her. You knew you wanted to cuddle and reassure your baby, but that may have been impossible because of the baby's constant medical care. Amelia recalled being so caught up in the medical and ethical emergencies surrounding her son John's premature birth that she felt she spent more time on the medical issues and crisis than on just loving her baby. 'There were so many decisions to be made,' Amelia said. 'I know I was protecting our baby's rights, but I spent so much time talking to the neonatologist and I wish I had spent it talking to John instead.'

If you were the mother of a critically ill baby who was transferred to a different hospital for special medical care before dying, the separation this imposed between you and your baby was especially wrenching. If your recovery was without complication, your hospital may have discharged you early so you could be with the baby. This time with your child may have been extremely meaningful to you, as it was for Rose, whose baby lived only twenty-three hours. 'I knew he was dying,' she said. 'But it made me feel better to be with him, to know at least I had done that for him.'

If you could not leave the hospital and your baby had to be transferred, you faced an unavoidable separation from your infant, which may have made you feel you had literally abandoned your baby. An experienced neonatologist suggests a number of practical measures that can help in this situation. After the baby's urgent medical problems have been attended to, he recommends the mother see and touch her infant before the transfer and suggests she keep a photograph of the baby with her. He advises the nursery staff to give her the name of a contact person she can call at any time for information about the baby's condition. The baby's father and grandparents should be encouraged to visit the baby as frequently as they wish and to describe the infant's condition to the mother. These measures are designed to allow the mother a feeling of connection to her baby, in spite of their separation.

Because of the emotional, physical, and even financial strains of caring for a critically ill baby, you may have struggled with a feeling of relief when your baby died. Although this is a normal response under the circumstances, it can be troubling, especially if you were unprepared to feel this way. Try to share this difficult emotion with your partner or with other understanding adults so you can gain the perspective you need to forgive yourself ultimately and move on with your life.

Causes of Newborn Death

Premature delivery and low birth weight from any number of complications are the primary causes of neonatal death, although with medical advances, the survival rate is always improving. Birth defects such as heart and kidney problems are frequently implicated in the death of a newborn baby. Maternal conditions or illnesses such as the group B streptococcus microorganism can also precipitate newborn death.

Complicated labour and deliveries used to be more frequently cited as factors in newborn death; however, with the increased technology used in antenatal care and labour monitoring, such deaths are now more rare. If a newborn death occurs from a complicated delivery, it is usually because the baby or the mother was sick during the pregnancy or because the oxygen supply was inhibited by a rare complication during labour.

Once you and your partner have suffered the death of a newborn baby, it is important that you try to discover the cause as quickly as possible. If the birth was premature, a maternal condition should be investigated and, if at all possible, corrected. If your baby showed signs of chromosomal or genetic abnormalities, a full autopsy and analysis of the baby's tissues should be undertaken. You may also want to consult a genetic specialist before embarking on another pregnancy.

If your baby died from asphyxia, or lack of oxygen, during labour and delivery, or if your baby was carried past the due date, you should inquire about tests that can monitor the baby's growth and health during your next pregnancy. These tests include scans, maternal blood tests, fetal monitoring which can all pick up signs of potential problems. However, these causes of newborn death are far less likely to be repeated in a subsequent pregnancy than other causes related to maternal health or genetic problems.

Emotional Aftermath of Newborn Death

As angry and cheated as you feel following your newborn's death, you probably cherish the brief memories you have of your child, discovering solace in having known your baby, even for a short time. 'In my darkest hours,' admitted Wendy, 'I was still grateful for the fact that at least I had two weeks with my daughter.'

You may be able to focus on some aspect of your baby's life that is positive and meaningful to you. Lisa's anencephalic daughter, who was expected to die within a few minutes following delivery, eventually lived for several hours. 'I think about my daughter,' marvelled Lisa, 'and how much she wanted to live – eight full hours! She was a real fighter! I loved her for that.' Her husband, Adam, felt that even in their daughter's short life, she must have known how much her parents really cared for her, loved her, and wanted her. 'That knowledge gave us something to cling to,' he admitted. 'The fact that she knew we held her and tried to comfort her as best we could gave us great comfort, too.'

You may worry about losing memories of your baby because they are so fleeting and fragile. Holding on to some tangible keepsakes – a journal, a cot blanket, or a toy – can be important. If you have photographs, you might put them in an album or a special picture frame.

Amelia put one of her baby's photographs in a magnetic frame on her fridge, where she could look at it whenever she was in the kitchen. 'I loved having her there,' said Amelia, 'and I loved having people ask about her picture. It helped break the ice a lot after she died when people came to visit and weren't sure of what to say.'

You may struggle to find some meaning to your sorrow in an attempt to give your baby's brief life purpose and dignity. After Amelia's first two babies died from prematurity, she gave birth to Jacob, who lived. Her suffering prompted her to reflect on the legacy of all her children:

> I keep asking myself why negative learnings are always so powerful. I think our losses have made me and my husband different people. I think and I hope that in terms of responding to other people in crisis situations we can do a better job because of our tragedies.
>
> The losses have made us not take anything for granted. Last summer there was a beautiful warm night, and the three of us – Charles, Jacob in his buggy, and I – went out for a walk after dinner. For us that walk together in the warmth of the evening was more pleasurable than if we had spent hundreds of pounds on some wonderful holiday. We have started placing more value on things that to others might be considered pretty mundane.

Wendy strongly believed that her daughter had been born for some positive purpose, even though her life had been so brief:

> If I felt Samantha served the purpose of only bringing hatred and anger into my life, I couldn't take it. I am more compassionate to people who suffer losses now that I have had my own. If I felt too sorry for myself, I couldn't do this for others. Samantha came to bring good into our lives, not bad. I do believe that.

What Can Help You Following a Stillbirth or Newborn Death

Stillbirth and newborn death create particular grieving difficulties. You had committed a great deal of time to the pregnancy and may have been totally unprepared for this tragic outcome. The birth became an end instead of a beginning, a sad occasion instead of a happy one.

Here are some suggestions to help you begin to grieve your loss:

- Try to find out as much as possible about what might have caused your baby's death. The more information you have, the better able you will be to grasp what has happened and plan for a future pregnancy.
- If you gave birth to an ill newborn, try to understand and accept any feelings of relief – and consequent guilt – you might experience after your infant's death. These are natural reactions to your loss and should lessen with time.
- However blameless, you may feel somehow responsible for your tragedy. Try to let go of this guilt; your sorrow is great enough without the burden of self-blame. It is important to focus on the fact that you cared for your baby and wanted the best for your child. Do your best to accept medical decisions you were forced to make quickly and without much preparation.
- Friends and family may attempt to pressure you into decisions such as whether to have a funeral for the baby or to dismantle the baby's room. Try to do what feels right for you and helps you to grieve and plan for your future.

CHAPTER 8

PRENATAL DIAGNOSIS AND ABORTION: THE BURDEN OF CHOICE

Our family was ready to go out for dinner when the obstetrician called. I could hear in her voice that she had bad news. I felt like I was in a tunnel; it was like a bad dream. I started screaming, right there in front of my husband and the kids. I had to wait two weeks before I had the abortion. The baby was kicking. I thought I would lose my mind.

ELAINE

When antenatal diagnosis revealed that your unborn baby was impaired, the discovery was devastating and probably created a crisis for you and your partner. If you had never resolved what you would do in this situation, you had to decide quickly; even if you had previously decided to end an impaired pregnancy, you still had to review and reconfirm this choice. You may have urgently turned to your health care providers – genetic counsellor, obstetrician, or paediatrician – for information, guidance, and help in your tragic and bewildering circumstances.

Some couples feel sure of their decision to end an impaired pregnancy. They know genetic testing poses certain risks, and are only willing to undergo the procedure because they would choose to have an abortion if abnormalities were found. 'This pregnancy was not meant to be,' one woman said. 'Aborting an impaired child is helping nature take its course.'

Other parents feel abortion is necessary due to the stigma and hardships both the disabled child and the family would endure in our culture. There are couples who have a clear sense of their personal limitations. Some parents are deeply concerned about their marriage not surviving the care of a handicapped child or the burden that would be placed on their other children in the future as the couple ages.

But for many parents, it is dreadful to choose between aborting a wanted but defective baby or giving birth to an impaired child. Ever since advances in medical technology created this dilemma, philosophers and religious leaders, as well as hospital ethics advisory boards worldwide, have been grappling with this agonizing choice. And even these experts have been unable to produce any uniform laws or guidelines. It is understandable if parents feel the right or best course of action is unclear and worry that they will pay a terrible price with either decision.

Your decision may have been further complicated by the fact that sometimes tests can diagnose a disorder but cannot indicate the severity of the impairment. This is true of Down's Syndrome, the disorder most commonly tested for and diagnosed. A child with this condition could be only mildly retarded, with minor physical problems, or severely retarded, with serious ailments including heart, digestive, and respiratory problems or leukaemia. You may have felt able to raise a mildly impaired child, but not a child who would need frequent hospitalizations.

If you had to make a decision based on imprecise medical information, you were forced to gamble when the stakes were your unborn child and the quality of your family's future. Understandably, you may find the mourning period that follows especially difficult. However blameless you are, your pain may be compounded by guilt, because you produced an impaired child and you ended the pregnancy. 'It's a double taboo,' commented one father. 'First, people think something is wrong with you because your baby was defective. Then they look down on you for having an abortion.'

Preparing for Antenatal Testing and Receiving the Results

Like many couples who receive an abnormal antenatal diagnosis, your tests may have been given without any counselling or preparation for a problematic outcome. You may not have seriously considered the possibility of a problem being detected, so you may not have weighed your options before the diagnosis came in. 'I looked around the waiting room before my amniocentesis, wondering what poor soul was going to get bad news,' recalled Elaine, who received a diagnosis of Down's Syndrome from her test. 'I never dreamed it would be me.'

Many genetic counsellors consider counselling prior to antenatal diagnosis an essential patient service. Counselling can help expectant parents carefully consider the implications of having or not having the tests. Parents should be informed about problems that may be detected and encouraged to think about what course of action they would take if this were to occur. The counsellor can arrange in advance the time and place to notify the couple in the event a problem is found – for example, at home in the evening when they are together, rather than at work.

If logistically possible, parents may want to schedule an appointment in advance so they receive either positive or negative test results in person. This prevents them from worrying that each time the phone rings, it could be the news they dread. If a problem is found and the parents do receive the news by phone, a meeting should be scheduled immediately in recognition of the urgency of the situation. A helpful counsellor conveys respect for the couple's personal values and religious beliefs and has referral information for other resources at hand. Should the parents decide to have an abortion, the genetic counsellor can make the appointment for them and call a few weeks later to see how they are doing.

Parents need help in thinking and talking about how they would feel living with the consequences of their choice, as well as the support or disapproval they may receive from those close to them. Aaron found his discussion with a medical geneticist about his unborn baby's Down's Syndrome very helpful:

> She explained the condition and the range of disability we might find. She told us about all our options and was really impartial. She said some people keep babies with Down's Syndrome. She told us about a special school for these kids we could visit. She said we could also place the child for adoption.
>
> She asked another very significant question. She knew we were feeling upset and guilty, but wondered what it would have been like for us had we not had the testing and had learned of the baby's problems at birth. We knew we would have been devastated, and that painful as the test results were, they allowed us an important choice.

Aaron and his wife found that this approach to counselling enabled them to learn the facts and hear each other's feelings and opinions. They discovered they were in agreement about terminating the pregnancy and supported each other's decision. The careful review of the known facts, the unknown variables, and the options available to them enabled them to make what they felt was an informed choice.

Unfortunately, many couples do not have access to a trained genetic counsellor, medical geneticist, or doctor knowledgeable in this specialized counselling process to help them sort through both the facts of the diagnosis and the difficult choices they face. Although their obstetrician recommends antenatal testing, when the results show a problem and the couple looks for compassionate help, it may not be forthcoming.

Hilary and Derek had suffered from infertility and were elated when they finally conceived, only to learn from antenatal testing that their unborn baby had Down's Syndrome. While in agreement about ending the pregnancy, they were distraught, and Hilary felt their doctor's response only added to their trauma:

> I called the clinic that had done the amniocentesis and was told my GP already had the results. I knew there was a problem, since they wouldn't tell me the outcome. I called my GP's surgery right away, from work. Evidently, the least senior doctor in the practice had been told to speak with me. He told me the results over the phone, and I had to drive to his surgery and meet my husband there. It's a wonder I didn't get in a car crash on the way over!
>
> First he kept us waiting for twenty-five minutes, with all these other pregnant women. Then, when he met with us, he was very clinical and cold. He told us about all the possible anomalies a baby with Down's Syndrome might have, in addition to the mental retardation. My husband tried to tell him we had decided to have an abortion, but he just kept on talking. He told us it was a boy, but we really didn't want to know the sex.
>
> The worst part was when he told us he wasn't sure he agreed with people having an abortion. At this point I really blew up! My doctor had strongly recommended the amniocentesis. I asked him why he was in a practice where people have this test if he was going to tell us not to have an abortion! He admitted he had not personally come to grips with this.

The crisis that began when you received the test results continued while you awaited the procedure, especially if the diagnosis was made after you could feel the baby's movements. 'Once you get the results,' one woman awaiting an abortion put it, 'every day your baby moves, you are dying inside.'

You deserved clear information about your unborn child's condition and respect for your decision. You needed caregivers who had come to terms with these difficult issues themselves so they could help you by listening carefully to your questions and discussing your concerns.

Your Hospital Stay

However secure you and your partner might have felt in your decision to end an impaired pregnancy, you may have been unprepared for the physical and emotional ordeal of the procedure. If you received abnormal results in the first trimester from the prenatal genetic test called chorionic villus sampling, or CVS, and decided to end the pregnancy, a standard D&C procedure was probably used. If you had the more common amniocentesis test performed in the second trimester, your doctor terminated the abnormal pregnancy either by inducing labour or less commonly by dilatation and evacuation (D&E).

Sometimes couples can choose which procedure to have, but often other factors determine the method, including how far advanced the pregnancy is and what medical facilities are available. If a severe problem is detected by scan, a definitive diagnosis of the baby's condition may be needed to determine the risk of the condition recurring in future pregnancies, and may only be possible following a specific procedure.

Many parents faced with the ordeal of ending a wanted but impaired pregnancy find it upsetting to have the procedure at a hospital where most abortions are for normal but unwanted pregnancies. There are good reasons why separate facilities are impractical, but couples need to know in advance if they are being sent to an abortion clinic. Aaron and his wife had no such preparation and were shocked by their experience:

> When I walked into the clinic with my wife, my first impulse was to turn around and walk out. The waiting room was full of teenage girls, who were presumably there to abort unplanned and unwanted pregnancies. And there we were, ending a pregnancy we had wanted so badly. We were in that waiting room for several hours. It was dreadful.

If labour is induced to end the pregnancy, the mother will go through full labour. This can be painful and emotionally exhausting even with medication, and can last from several hours to a day or so. A couple's experience of the birth may vary widely, depending on the hospital staff and the type of procedure. In most hospitals staff give the couple the choice of seeing and holding the baby, and discuss plans for a funeral or burial with them. Most parents choose at least one of these options when they are offered. If you were not given a choice and wish you had said goodbye to your baby, try to remember that it was the staff's responsibility to offer you this opportunity, not yours to ask.

Hospital staff sometimes encourage the couple to make decisions about seeing the baby or having a burial prior to the abortion, painful though that may be. The alternative is to decide quickly right after the procedure, when the woman is often in a haze of medication.

Although hospital staff are sometimes reluctant to show parents a malformed baby, it is important for a couple to see their child, but it helps if a caregiver prepares the parents beforehand by describing any visible abnormalities and reassuring them they did nothing to cause the condition. Parents can be fearful of their baby's appearance and are relieved if the infant looks normal because the impairments are internal or mental. On the other hand, seeing visible defects can help to validate a parent's decision to end the pregnancy.

If the baby's father cannot stay with the mother during the procedure, it is wise for her to bring a friend or relative with her for physical and emotional support, if at all possible. It is also important for medical staff and relatives to keep in mind that fathers feel the sense of loss as well and to include them in expressions of care and concern in the aftermath of the abortion.

What to Tell Your Children at Home

If you have children at home, you may want to plan how to discuss the loss with them, a difficult task while you are coping with your own distress. You may find yourself struggling to explain the situation to your youngsters in a way that is as truthful as possible without being too upsetting.

Many parents experience difficulty when trying to explain an abortion to children old enough to know their mother was pregnant but too young to grasp the issues involved in ending an abnormal pregnancy. Most children react to this kind of loss as they would to a spontaneous loss. They may feel angry and disappointed that the expected baby is not coming home and can worry that playing rough with their mother, or harbouring feelings of jealousy, caused the loss.

With children from the ages of three to about ten, it is best to give a partial explanation without telling them the abortion was your decision. Instead, you may want to say the baby didn't grow properly from the very beginning or that the pregnancy miscarried, without saying that you had an abortion. Telling a small child you ended a pregnancy because the baby was abnormal or sick could make your youngster worry that if *he* gets sick, or has something wrong with *him*, you might get rid of him, too.

As you prepare to explain this loss to your children, keep in mind that as they grow older they will probably question you about it again. You may find it helpful initially to include known facts about the baby's abnormalities, such as heart or chromosomal defects, so you have a foundation for a franker discussion in the future.

With preteens and teenagers, who are probably aware of antenatal testing and know the facts about abortion, you face a more difficult task. It is hard to tell an adolescent who is inevitably struggling with his own imperfections that you aborted a 'less than perfect' child.

You may find it helpful to share with your adolescent children your own thoughts and feelings about the suffering of the baby or the sacrifices required by the family when a handicapped child is born. You might acknowledge that this was a difficult decision for you, with no easy answer, and then be guided by your adolescent's questions.

If your children are very young, or if you have others after the abortion, it will probably be important to tell them at some time about the antenatal diagnosis and your decision to end the pregnancy. This may be necessary when young children reach adolescence or when grown children need information about the family's medical history.

Chapter 12, 'Helping Your Children at Home,' includes a complete discussion of ways you can talk with your children about the loss, to help you understand their worries, and to help them cope with their own sadness.

Your Emotional Recovery

Your choice to end your impaired pregnancy can have a painful emotional aftermath, as it entails losses on many levels. You are mourning the terminated pregnancy and you are also grieving for the wished-for, healthy child you did not conceive. The trauma may be intensified because your loss was in part by choice and not only by chance.

Although you may have ended the pregnancy to spare your child incapacity, illness, and anguish, your decision to have an abortion can undermine your identity as a loving, nurturing parent.

Even if you feel certain you made the right decision, you may occasionally wonder what your life would be like if you had made the other choice. The burden of this decision and its accompanying guilt are terrible, and contribute to the suffering that follows this kind of loss. As one father put it, 'Everybody feels bad for you and says you made the right decision. But *you* made the decision – and *you* have to live with it.'

Dr Dion Donnai and a group of colleagues in Manchester, have conducted studies that indicate that both women and men are more depressed after they choose to end an impaired pregnancy than after having a spontaneous loss or aborting a normal but unwanted pregnancy. You may feel singled out and stigmatized, especially if you do not know anyone else who has experienced this kind of loss. You may fear criticism and only inform your friends and colleagues that you had a loss, without saying the baby was defective or that you were forced to make an agonizing choice.

One mother who told friends she had a spontaneous loss rather than an abortion had a friend remark to her that the loss 'was God's will.' 'Well, yes,' she thought, 'the first part, the disability, was. The second part was my decision.' The isolation you may feel, and the inability to speak freely of your ordeal, can worsen your depression.

Parents, especially mothers, faced with this type of loss often show intense emotional symptoms that may persist from three months to a year or more. 'I had nightmares, terrible headaches, and no energy for anything,' Lily recalled. 'I dreamed that my children were drowning in front of me and I couldn't save them.' Elaine admitted that she was irritable and tearful for months. 'I started feeling better,' she recalled, 'then it got worse again, as the anniversary approached.' She noted that she had been unable to lose the extra weight from her pregnancy in reaction to her psychological trauma. 'I'm punishing myself for having time for myself,' she explained, 'instead of caring for a sick baby.'

Men as well as women suffer from depression after this kind of loss. One father was left particularly bitter, feeling that the basic strivings of life, such as raising a healthy family, were unattainable. Another man who had been through years of infertility and had then aborted a baby with Down's Syndrome was deeply shaken. He found it difficult to be around children and gave up some friends and favourite recreational activities because he knew children would be present.

There is also a high incidence of marital separation among couples during the stressful aftermath of ending an impaired pregnancy. The fact that men and women grieve differently after an abortion, just as they do following a spontaneous loss, contributes to the couple's distress. Although marital stress often persists for many months, follow-up studies have shown that most couples eventually reunite.

You may, however, find that a stronger bond is forged between you. When Derek and Hilary ended a pregnancy because of a Down's Syndrome diagnosis, the devotion her husband demonstrated throughout their ordeal made a lasting impression on Hilary:

> We are closer as a result of the loss. I never realized how much I meant to my husband or how dependable he was. I didn't know the extent of how good he was to me until all this happened.

Many factors can affect how you manage in the early weeks and months after you end an impaired pregnancy, including your personality, the strength of your marriage, and the availability of other sources of support and comfort. Both you and your partner will need patient, understanding family and friends, and possibly professional support as well, as you endure the sad aftermath of this difficult loss.

Finding the Support You Need

You may find that reaching out for support from others is key to your recovery after this emotional ordeal. You must choose your listeners with care, however, because while some people may welcome this opportunity to be supportive, others may not be sympathetic to your decision. If you tell compassionate family and friends what the loss meant to you, describing the grief and turmoil you are going through, you may receive genuine sympathy and concern in return.

This was true for Lily, who had one healthy child followed by two abortions after antenatal diagnosis indicated severe genetic problems both times. She was very depressed, especially after the second abortion, and wondered what to tell her friends. 'In the end I just told them the truth,' she admitted. 'I had no energy to lie, or hide it, or say it was a miscarriage. And people were wonderful.'

Elaine also reached out to friends when she conceived a baby with Down's Syndrome. She felt upset, guilty, and depressed when she and her husband decided to end the pregnancy, emotions that only intensified when her husband didn't want to talk about the loss at all. Elaine found that she needed the outlet of friends to whom she could say, 'I'm going nuts today!' As she explained, 'It really helped to know my friends were there for me.'

Both of you may find psychotherapy helpful, either together or individually, so you can unburden yourselves without worrying about bringing up a subject friends and relatives may feel is taboo. The opportunity to talk with an understanding professional can lessen your distress during the difficult aftermath of your loss.

Like many couples, you may feel that your hurt is healed only after a subsequent, healthy child is born or adopted. You may discover that you are more open to life experiences that give you a greater perspective on your tragedy. Hilary, an occupational therapist, said her work with accident victims helped her cope with her abortion. As she explained, 'I know from my job that life isn't fair to any of us and that there are others a lot worse off than me.'

You might find you only gradually come to terms with the decision you made by honestly facing your personal, psychological, and family limitations. Accepting how difficult raising an impaired child might have been for you and your partner can help alleviate your guilt.

Rebecca's antenatal diagnosis had revealed a rare chromosomal disorder that would probably have caused mental retardation and mental illness. Her husband could not cope with the prospect of a mentally impaired child, and Rebecca realized she felt the same way:

> I had to face the fact that someone else in the same situation would have chosen to have the baby. There are some things I don't totally like about myself. I have limitations. But this is who I am.

Parents tend to reproach themselves less, and to adjust better following their abortion, if they had experienced firsthand the impairment that was diagnosed. Some adults who grew up with an impaired family member may not want to put themselves through the same suffering again, nor want to inflict it on their child. They also may not want their other children to be burdened later in life by having to care for a handicapped sibling.

One doctor spoke of a couple who had watched their first baby deteriorate and die from Gaucher disease, a progressive neurological disorder. When the couple's next baby was found to have the same condition, the father remarked:

After seeing what the first baby went through, there was nothing to think about in deciding to abort. It is hard to feel guilt after seeing our first baby suffer.

Perhaps because of the unique psychological and moral dilemmas involved in ending an impaired pregnancy, there are few pregnancy loss support groups in the UK geared specifically for couples who experience this kind of tragedy. Some support groups for spontaneous losses have sensitive and tolerant members who welcome couples who have terminated a pregnancy after an abnormal prenatal diagnosis. But couples who faced a choice and have to live with their decision may find these issues are not addressed adequately. They also may worry about encountering a judgmental attitude from group members personally opposed to abortion.

Parents who do have access to a support group designed for couples who have endured this ordeal describe it as enormously beneficial. Hilary attended such a group after enduring years of infertility and then aborting an impaired pregnancy. Although she was clear about her decision, the diagnosis seemed particularly cruel after waiting so long for her 'miracle baby.' Hilary was surprised at how much the group helped her:

Before I went into the group, I thought no one in the world could be as badly off. Then we learned that another couple in the group had also been through years of infertility before their loss. Even people in the group with healthy children at home were just as devastated.

The group helped us to get out the things we were not willing to face. We chose to have an abortion because I know Down's Syndrome children can be born with physical as well as mental handicaps and that they can suffer greatly. And we had to look at how we would care for a handicapped child when we were sixty. But I didn't want to accept that part of my decision was selfish, that I didn't want a less-than-perfect child.

Then other couples said they blamed themselves for not being strong enough to deal with an abnormal child. When they said this, it was like a dagger through my heart, because I knew it was true for me, too. I cried for two solid days, but I had to face my guilt. Those feelings are there, and if you don't get them out, they eat away at you.

I would recommend this group for anyone, even for a very shy person. I don't usually see myself as a group person, but it was highly therapeutic.

If a support group does not exist in your area, consider asking your doctor or genetic counsellor to put you in touch with another parent who has been through a similar loss, with that parent's permission. Couples who have gone through this difficult loss are often willing to talk with others in the same situation.

It takes time and support for you gradually to integrate the tragedy of your loss into your life. You may find that ending an impaired pregnancy has changed you and that in some ways you will never be the same. 'I think about it every day, even just for a second,' one woman remarked. 'But life has to go on.' Grieving your loss, and the normal baby who never was, will help you eventually shift your focus to other, positive aspects of your life.

As time passes, and you get some distance from your tragedy, you may feel your decision was right for you and your family, but you might still deeply regret that you were forced to choose. 'I don't feel bad about the decision,' one woman reasoned. 'I'm just sorry I had to be put in that situation.'

What Can Help After You End an Impaired Pregnancy

You may find the process of emotional recovery after ending an impaired pregnancy to be a long one. Although in no way at fault for the abnormality, you may feel you have failed as a parent, both for having produced an impaired child and for having an abortion. Your memory of the abortion and of being forced into an active decision can stay with you for a long time.

You also carry the special burden of having to decide how much to tell relatives and friends about your loss. If you decide to keep the fact of the abortion private, you may feel even more depressed as you find yourself cut off from potential sources of support.

Here are some suggestions to help you cope with the special difficulties associated with your loss:

- Once you decide to end your pregnancy, try to be well informed about any choices of procedure you may have. Find out in advance what the procedure you will have is like. Be sure both you and your partner are there together, or arrange for another support person to stay with you during the procedure.

- If you missed the opportunity to see and hold your baby and regret this, try not to blame yourself because hospital staff did not give you these options.
- If you feel the need for a ritual following your loss, see also Chapter 10 and Appendix B.
- If you have other children, you may want to decide with your partner how you will discuss the loss with them. If you have questions about this, a hospital social worker or qualified psychotherapist can advise you. See also Chapter 12, 'Helping Your Children at Home.'
- You may face an especially difficult time at home after your loss, so try to find caring people to help you through the initial grieving period. Speak with understanding family and friends, join a support group, or ask your obstetrician or genetic counsellor to put you in touch with another couple who has had a similar loss. Counselling can be a vital help, especially if support from family and friends is lacking.

SECTION III
The Response of Others

As personal as your pregnancy loss may seem, you share it not only with your partner but with many others as well. From the medical staff member who first tells you of your loss to your dearest relatives and friends who attempt to console you, other people will have an impact on your ability to acknowledge your loss and handle your grief.

Your capacity to cope with your loss depends greatly on how those around you react to your sorrow. Some may say the right thing and provide comfort and solace when you need them most. Others may inadvertently utter the wrong words or offer inappropriate advice, making you feel alienated and hurt when you deserve to feel accepted and soothed.

The following chapters address these issues and can help you manage both your sorrow and your anger when you feel you have not been treated compassionately or fairly. You will also read about how to help your children at home deal with your loss and how grandparents can learn to cope when their child loses a pregnancy.

CHAPTER 9

MEDICAL CARE WHEN YOU LOSE YOUR PREGNANCY

In the aftermath of your pregnancy loss, you may realize the medical care you received has a lasting impact on your emotional recovery. The ability of medical staff to go beyond concern for your physical well-being and to acknowledge your grief probably affected your expression of sorrow at the time of your loss and your capacity to grieve now. If the medical staff was properly trained in bereavement counselling, they supported your expression of sorrow and guided you in anticipating your emotional state in the difficult weeks and months following your loss.

If your loss was mismanaged by a medical professional – whether a midwife, obstetrician, or a radiographer undertaking a scan – you may have been further traumatized and your mourning impeded.

Learning About Your Loss

You will probably remember forever the way you learned about your pregnancy loss. At this personal and tragic moment, you deserved to be told the truth directly by a compassionate medical caregiver who acknowledged your loss. If you received thoughtful treatment, you were probably better able to focus on the reality of your tragedy and to begin grieving appropriately.

Gloria recalled how important it was for her to have her doctor and midwife present when her baby's death *in utero* was confirmed. 'My doctor got teary-eyed when she saw the ultrasound, and the midwife was visibly moved, too,' Gloria recalled. 'It meant a lot to me for them to be there and to show that kind of feeling.'

If your doctor was sensitive to your situation, he probably told you of the loss when both you and your partner were present. The doctor respected your need to absorb the news and to ask questions as well as to have private time with your partner. However, you may have learned of your loss in a way that added to your distress. This is more likely to have occurred if you were cared for by medical personnel you did not know, such as a partner in your doctor's practice, or casualty staff.

Carmen went to casualty after her midwife detected a problem when she was thirty-one weeks pregnant:

> No one talked to me or looked at me. The doctors talked among themselves, saying they could not find a heartbeat. Nobody told me the baby was dead; no one actually said the word. I suppose they thought I would guess. Then they left me in the hall in a wheelchair, crying.

If you experienced an early pregnancy loss, you may have found your doctor not only failed to acknowledge your grief but also actively minimized your sorrow. Many doctors have the medical perspective that a miscarriage is a normal part of a woman's overall reproductive experience and is often followed by a healthy pregnancy and delivery. This view, as well as your doctor's wish to protect you and himself from sadness, can also make him downplay your genuine grief.

Annette had a miscarriage that her doctor presumed was due to a blighted ovum, but his medical reasssurances did not diminish the sadness she felt at losing her baby:

> He told me that it happened for the best, that it wasn't a healthy pregnancy anyway. But I wasn't comforted by those comments at all. I was nurturing and carrying a baby I loved, even if it was only for a short time. Then to be told my loss was for the best because the baby wasn't healthy, good, or perfect seemed to be an excuse to tell me I shouldn't be sad.

Your unborn baby's death may have been confirmed by a nurse or doctor you had never met before. You may have seen for yourself on the ultrasound screen that there was no heartbeat, or received the news of your pregnancy loss from the person you didn't know who conducted the test. Perhaps you had one of those radiographers who would not tell you the outcome, but left you guessing and frantic while they conveyed the results to your doctor, who then told you the news in person or by phone. You may have preferred to hear the news directly from the radiographer without having to wait.

At such a difficult time, even small gestures of concern are remembered and appreciated. When Ellen's scan confirmed her third miscarriage, she left the examining room visibly upset. 'The radiographer followed me out and asked if I was all right,' Ellen recalled. 'I wasn't all right, and there was nothing she could really do, but it meant a lot to me that she asked.'

In your sorrow, you may believe that your shock would have been lessened if your doctor had provided more information about pregnancy loss before your problem developed. If your loss occurred after you began childbirth classes, you may feel angry that your tutor never even alluded to such possibilities. Perhaps you assumed your pregnancy was safe as long as you kept your medical appointments, took good care of your health, and prepared properly for the birth.

Doctors and childbirth educators can feel in a bind because pregnant women and their partners generally do not want to hear about losses, nor do medical professionals want to cause needless worry. And there is probably nothing a caregiver could have said in way of preparation that would have diminished your sadness.

Some obstetricians do explain which symptoms might jeopardize a pregnancy or be warning signs of an impending loss and warrant immediate medical attention, such as a high fever, vaginal bleeding, or loss of amniotic fluid. Pregnant women who are given this kind of matter-of-fact information are more likely to become informed participants in all aspects of their antenatal care. While most do not imagine *their* pregnancy could end in loss, they know problems in pregnancy can occur, so that if they experience a loss they perceive it as a tragic event but not a bizarre one.

Your Hospital Care

All around I felt I was given the lowest priority because the baby had died. I told them I wanted an epidural for the delivery, but the anaesthetist arrived too late. The staff avoided me. They didn't seem to know what to do with me. I had to pester them to get injections to stop my milk before I went home.

CARMEN

I'll never forget when I went into the special care nursery where our daughter had been placed to live out her short life. The nurse asked me, 'How are you doing, Mum?' Tears streamed down my face. That meant so much to me. Nobody else at the hospital ever acknowledged the fact that I was a mum.

LISA

Although one in five pregnancies ends in a first-trimester miscarriage and about one in eighty deliveries results in a stillbirth or newborn death, many hospital obstetrical departments still lack bereavement services for parents who suffer a loss.

The field of obstetrics, in particular, is geared toward bringing new life into the world. When death occurs where new life is expected, untrained and unprepared obstetrical staff react with anxiety and helplessness, making it difficult for them to assist bereaved families. Staff members untrained in bereavement may respond to a pregnancy loss by avoiding the grieving parents because they don't know what to say, or because they are afraid the parents will only cry and become more upset, not realizing this is just what bereaved parents need permission to do.

The Stillbirth and Neonatal Death Society, however, has produced a booklet entitled 'Miscarriage, stillbirth and neonatal death; guidelines for professionals'. Endorsed by all the major professional bodies and associations, it aims to help professionals give parents who suffer pregnancy loss or infant death the quality of care that is appropriate in these difficult circumstances. The guidelines suggest that parents need help from hospital staff to express their love and say goodbye to their baby. If the loss occurs after the first trimester, parents may want mementos such as a picture, footprints, or a lock of hair. They should also be given the chance to see and hold their child. With any pregnancy loss, bereaved parents should have access to grief counselling, pastoral care, and options for rituals, as well as guidance on how to obtain relevant medical information following their tragedy.

Like many bereaved parents, you may fault yourself for not having requested these services. Given your emotional state after your loss, you could not have taken the initiative in requesting appropriate care. Clinical studies have repeatedly shown that when hospital staff do not offer bereavement services, most parents do not ask for the care they need and do not receive it. It is the hospital's responsibility to train staff in bereavement protocols so patients are provided with this important service.

If you are a mother whose loss posed a danger to your life, such as ectopic pregnancy or premature separation of the placenta, you may have found that hospital staff ignored your emotional response to your loss. The medical emergency shifted the focus of concern from the pregnancy to you.

Doctors and nurses are, after all, primarily responsible for the medical care of their patients, not their emotional well-being, especially in life-and-death circumstances. But like many bereaved mothers, you may have felt the need for some simple acknowledgment of your loss, even in the face of a medical crisis.

Tracy felt that the grief she experienced following emergency surgery for an ectopic pregnancy was completely overlooked:

> I think the medical staff should be more sensitive to the woman's need to mourn. They should acknowledge that there was indeed a loss, even if they feel she should be grateful simply to be alive. I *was* grateful, of course, but I was also tremendously sad because I was mourning the loss of a baby I wanted so badly.

As a bereaved mother there are many specific issues about your medical care that you bore alone. The location where you were placed in the hospital for your care probably had a profound effect on you. If you were cared for on the labour ward, you probably heard other mothers giving birth to healthy babies, which was undoubtedly distressing for you. However, if you were in a surgical ward, with cancer and other postoperative patients, you may have found yourself to be the nurses' lowest priority. You may have been virtually uncared for during your labour, and your need to be comforted after your loss was probably completely overlooked.

Martha was two months pregnant when she started bleeding profusely. Her doctor sent her to the hospital, where she was put in a room on a surgical ward.

> I was left unattended for hours. No one came in to check on me, or hand me a bedpan. At 4:00 A.M. I passed the baby. A nurse took it and was going to throw it away until I told her I wanted my doctor to examine it. She got a jar and put it on my nightstand. That was upsetting, too.
>
> During my two-day hospital stay, I cried constantly. Someone could have said, 'Do you want to talk?' or 'Is there anything you need?' I got nothing.

Some hospitals avoid this problem by treating women who are showing signs of pregnancy loss on the antenatal ward where nurses may be more aware of their physical and emotional needs. But when an unborn baby is known to have died already, the mother may be left unattended here as well. 'In part this is because the nurses don't have the health of the baby to worry about,' one midwife pointed out, 'and in part it's because they don't know what to say.'

Where you were transferred for recovery after your loss also depended on hospital facilities and policy. Your hospital may have automatically transferred you out of the nursing mothers area to a gynaecology ward, where you may have been more comfortable away from new mothers and babies. If the nursing staff and other caregivers were trained to care for your special needs, you probably felt emotionally protected as well.

After Carla suffered a pregnancy loss at twenty-six weeks in the delivery room, she was transferred to the gynaecology ward, where she found the nursing care to be extremely helpful:

> The nurses held my hand and were sympathetic. A couple of them gave me and my husband their phone numbers and told us to call anytime we wanted someone to talk to. One nurse gave me something to read on pregnancy loss. She said, 'I know you can't look at it now. Take it; it will help you later.' The social worker was wonderful as well. She came to see me twice and gave me information about support groups.

The value of medical staff having bereavement training and established procedures for handling pregnancy loss becomes painfully clear in its absence. Without guidelines, details are bound to be forgotten.

Laura went into labour when only twenty-three weeks pregnant and knew her baby could not survive. She delivered on the gynaecology ward without seeing her baby, whom the nurse quickly removed. The next morning her doctor came to see Laura and her husband. He was compassionate, and gently but firmly encouraged the couple to see their infant, but he neglected to swaddle the tiny baby, departing from the SANDS professional guidelines.

> He brought her into my room and with gloved hands, removed her from the surgical container she had been in. He held her little body for us to see.
>
> I cried, realizing that she was so perfect. I cried realizing that her death was so final and I understood none of it. Later, months later, I would cry at this thoughtlessness – seeing our daughter lifted like a laboratory specimen, dripping wet, from a container filled with saline solution.

Your need for special emotional care from staff continued after your loss.

Contact with a nurse, social worker, or your obstetrician, who allowed time for you to review your loss in detail, may have been extremely helpful. Both you and your partner needed a chance to share your feelings with staff and one another.

Special Considerations with Stillbirth and Newborn Death

Our baby was born very prematurely when I was five months pregnant. We knew she wouldn't survive. I didn't see her, and I didn't know if it was okay to ask to see her. I finally asked if it was a boy or a girl. I never asked if she was alive, and I never asked to hold her. I was haunted by this long afterward.

RUTH

I stayed up the entire time Michelle lived. I couldn't bear the thought of going to sleep during any of her life because it was going to be so short. I didn't want to miss a single moment. The staff were wonderful. They had a room next to the neonatal ward where my husband and I could stay with Michelle. She died in our arms.

GAIL

As a mother, there were many crucial decisions you had to confront once you were hospitalized. If you laboured with a baby who was stillborn or not expected to live, you had to choose whether to take pain medication during delivery. You may have been torn by the desire to experience the entire process of giving birth and the wish to be free from the physical pain of a hard, fruitless labour. 'Even knowing our daughter was going to die,' admitted Ruth, 'I still didn't want to have drugs and not be there for her. However brief her life was to be, I wanted to be her mummy every minute.'

If you remain troubled about your decision to take or avoid pain medication during delivery, try to accept that you made your best choice under severe stress or that your doctor took the decision out of your hands. You could not be expected to make reasoned decisions under these circumstances.

If your baby was stillborn or born seriously ill, staff may have encouraged you and your partner to see and hold your infant. Holding the baby and saying goodbye may have helped you express your love and begin to grieve, while missing this opportunity could leave a legacy of regret.

Medical staff trained in bereavement should have taken the initiative in helping you see your baby. Your first impulse may have been *not* to see your child because you were still in emotional shock, afraid of the baby's appearance, or so angry at the baby for dying.

When Hilary's premature twins died at birth, she relied on the hospital nurse for these unexpected decisions:

> We had a great nurse who realized our emotional state. She knew we wouldn't ask for a picture or to hold the babies. She brought the babies to us and encouraged us to hold them. Afterward we were both really grateful we did.

Part of the bereavement staff's role would have been to prepare you for your baby's appearance, including the infant's size, colouring, and other features, depending on the gestational age and the cause of your loss. Even if your child had visible malformations, as long as you knew what to expect, you probably focused on the positive aspects of your infant's appearance.

Before the nurse brought Lisa's anencephalic baby to her, she explained that a little knitted cap would be placed over the baby's improperly developed skull. She also gently told Lisa that the baby's eyes looked vacant. Seeing and holding her baby left an indelible yet positive impression on Lisa once she was properly prepared:

> I was able to tell my mother that her granddaughter was beautiful. She had beautiful long legs and arms, and she had my mouth and nose. Only her eyes had that empty look. She was very small, but I was struck by her beauty.

The death of your baby was a loss for the entire family, not just for you and your partner. Your parents, siblings, and other children at home were all affected. If your hospital policy was enlightened, they may have allowed relatives and close friends to share with you in seeing and holding your baby.

Hospital staff may also have offered you the option of naming your child. Many parents do not know this is possible; yet, when told they may name their babies, most do so. If you named your baby, this acknowledged the importance of the infant and can help you and loved ones to talk about the baby and grieve your loss.

You may have wished to keep mementoes such as a baby blanket, cot card, identification bracelet, or lock of hair. Hopefully, the medical staff offered these keepsakes in a way that helped you feel at ease about accepting them and did not make you wonder if you were morbid for wanting evidence of your baby's existence and identity.

You may also have wanted a photograph of your baby especially if you were not able to bring your own camera to the delivery room. Hospitals usually use instant cameras so they can give parents their pictures immediately and can take additional photographs if necessary. Either Polaroid or a good film reproduction lab can make copies from the original photograph, even without a negative.

If your picture was taken by a staff member trained in bereavement, the baby was carefully cleaned and wrapped in a blanket. It is also suggested that a second picture, of the uncovered baby, also be taken, especially if the mother was sedated during delivery. This second picture can remind you of details about your baby's appearance you may not recall from the delivery room.

If a photograph was taken and you did not want to bring it home, it was probably placed in your medical record. You can request it later, even weeks or months after your infant's death, when you may need it to help you remember and grieve the baby who never came home.

If you suffered a stillbirth or newborn death, you were probably asked whether you wanted to have an autopsy performed. Some parents do not believe this procedure will yield significant information and choose not to have an autopsy. However, if the doctor does not know the cause of your baby's death and can not therefore issue a death certificate, the death has to be reported to a coroner who will arrange for a postmortem. You cannot withhold your consent for this.

Many parents do want an autopsy performed in order to clarify the diagnosis or the risk of a similar loss occurring in future pregnancies. The quesion itself, however, may have shocked you, bringing home so concretely the finality of your baby's death.

An autopsy is a detailed examination of the baby in which some surgery is necessary to remove tissues from internal organs for microscopic inspection. You can still have an open casket at a funeral if the autopsy is performed with this in mind. You will usually receive preliminary results within a couple of weeks; however, you may have to wait up to three months for a complete, written report.

An autopsy can be helpful for several reasons. You may question whether you did anything to contribute to the baby's death, a fear an autopsy can often dispel. In some cases an autopsy determines a specific cause of death, which gives you information about future risks and medical care. If the death was due to a cord accident or a problem with the placenta, but the baby's physical development was normal, you may be comforted, since the likelihood of a recurrence is quite low. You may also have consented to an autopsy in the hope that the information it yielded would help medical science and other babies in the future, allowing some good to come out of your tragedy.

You were probably faced with unexpected decisions about burial, cremation, or a religious service for your baby. A hospital social worker, nurse, or chaplain may have helped you review your options and make appropriate choices, or you may have received no assistance at all. Some parents are guided by religious laws, but you, like many others, may have made a rapid decision to have the hospital take care of cremation or burial and only later wished you had done more for your baby.

While you cannot undo the finality of some missed opportunities, such as not seeing your baby or having a burial, there are some experiences and choices you *can* alter, even after the fact. Regrets can add to your grief, so talking about them with a supportive person is a vital first step. If you did not have a ritual when the loss occurred, you can still name your baby and hold a memorial service to honour your child. Suggestions for rituals are discussed in Chapter 10, 'Finding Solace in Your Religion,' and in Appendix B.

Communication Among Medical Staff

All medical staff who came in contact with you and your partner should have been informed of your loss. If communication was lacking, staff may have made small mistakes that were nevertheless devastating, such as asking the mother of a stillborn baby if she was breast- or bottle-feeding.

Poor communication among medical staff may have had an equally harmful effect if you and your partner experienced an early loss. You may have received phone calls confirming an amniocentesis appointment, or had a visit from a community midwife after your due delivery date.

If you had undergone antenatal tests before your loss occurred, the hospital may have sent the results directly to you, with upsetting consequences. 'The day I came home from the hospital after losing my baby in the fifth month,' remembered Ruth, 'I got a call from the hospital lab saying the results of the amniocentesis were fine, that I was carrying a healthy baby girl.' If you had this experience, consider alerting your doctor so he can arrange for the laboratory to check with him before contacting patients in the future.

You and your partner may have been needlessly distressed if the mother was referred to specialized services, such as radiology, where doctors and technicians were unaware of your situation. Two weeks before her due date, Lisa learned her baby had a lethal malformation. She was referred for an X-ray to check on the baby's position for inducing labour, but the technician had not been informed of the diagnosis:

> She gave me a terrible time. She wouldn't do the X-ray because I was pregnant! She wanted me to sign something to release her of responsibility for the X-ray. I was so upset that the baby would not live, and having to fight with hospital staff was so cruel.

If you need to alert the hospital about your loss, you may want to ask a relative or friend to call for you to avoid being telephoned or having to make these difficult calls yourself. If hospital staff involved in your care were unaware of your loss, you may want to let the hospital know about this problem so they can correct their procedures for future patients. Suggestions for taking this kind of action are discussed later in this chapter.

Your Hospital Discharge and Follow-up Care

Before I left the hospital, no one said I might be depressed after a miscarriage. My hormones were going wild, my breasts hurt. I thought I was going nuts when the doctor pinched my cheek and said, 'You'll be fine.' I thought I wasn't supposed to be having these other feelings. I left the hospital so depressed, so empty, so hurt, I'm surprised I didn't have a nervous breakdown on the way home.

MARTHA

In addition to needing sensitive bereavement counselling while the mother was in the hospital, you and your partner deserved preparation for the stresses you faced when you returned home. If your caregivers were trained in bereavement, they may have assured you that your grief was normal and forewarned you that it might improve only gradually, over several weeks or months. They may have explained that husbands and wives can grieve quite differently. The staff may also have guided you on how to discuss the loss with other children at home, to minimize the youngsters' anxiety and allow them to grieve as well.

Bereavement services may have included written information about pregnancy loss and grief, as well as a list of appropriate bereavement support groups in your community. If you did not receive this information before going home, you may be able to obtain it through your hospital nursing or social work department. You might not be ready for this material right away, but it can be a lifeline in the difficult weeks and months ahead.

Because no one can absorb information well immediately after a loss, follow-up contact is usually needed. If your baby was in an intensive care unit before she died, neonatal staff you know personally may have given you the name of a doctor or nurse in the department to call if you wanted to talk or if you had questions after your baby's death.

Rose's full-term baby died of congenital defects one day after birth. Both the intensive care paediatrician and the surgeon who operated on her daughter gave Rose their phone numbers and made themselves available:

> We did call back a couple of times in the weeks after the death, with different questions. Once my husband called because he had given blood when the baby needed a transfusion. He had drunk a glass of wine beforehand and wondered if the wine in his system had harmed the baby. The doctor assured him this was not so.

This kind of follow-up, however, is unusual for departments other than the neonatal nursery. Few obstetricians routinely phone their patients after a pregnancy loss. As a bereaved parent, you may be hurt by this lack of contact, especially if your loss occurred late in the pregnancy. After months of regular appointments, you want to know your welfare remains important to your doctor, even though your baby died. Bess, who suffered a stillbirth shortly before her due date, felt her doctor should have remained involved after her loss:

> My doctor never called after my stillbirth. Someone called me from his surgery with a minor query; they didn't even mention the loss.
>
> It would have been a kind thing to do, to call one or two months later to see how I was managing. I had seen the doctor regularly for eight months. I felt he owed me a phone call.

Like most bereaved parents, contact with your doctor and hospital was probably limited to your follow-up visit or a meeting to review laboratory reports or autopsy results. Hopefully, your doctor saw you promptly, so you did not have a long wait in the company of pregnant women and new mothers.

Bereaved parents can need a number of special services from their doctor, including referrals for genetic counselling or a high-risk centre. A caring doctor will ask how the woman and her family are managing emotionally and may offer referral information on psychotherapy or support groups. Couples can be upset when their doctors fail to offer this information and might feel the physicians have done them a real disservice.

It took Leonard several phone calls to locate a support group in his area:

> It is criminal for doctors not to have in their surgery information about support groups, the name of a therapist and of counselling facilities. Patients should not have to go searching for this – they are dealing with enough as it is.

Unfortunately, many doctors do not ask after the rest of the family during the follow-up visit. Some do not mention the loss at all, or – even worse – do not remember it. Dr Stanford Bourne, an obstetrician, conducted a study of doctors' reactions to mothers who had a stillbirth and found their doctors tended not 'to know, notice, or remember anything about the patient who has had a stillbirth.' If this happened to you, it probably felt like the ultimate negation of your tragedy.

Carla went in for a postnatal check-up six weeks after her premature baby died. While she was being examined, the doctor asked her, 'How's the baby?' Carla, incredulous, said, 'Excuse me?' 'Oh, how is everything?' corrected her doctor. 'You're looking good, you look like you're recovering.' Carla changed doctors.

Some doctors shy away from discussing a loss with bereaved parents for fear of courting a lawsuit. In fact the opposite is probably true, that more litigation seems to result from poor interpersonal relations than from actual medical malpractice. You and your partner were probably quick to pick up on your doctor's reluctance to acknowledge your loss or to give you information frankly. This may have felt like a breach in the doctor-patient relationship that left you disillusioned with your care.

How You Can Improve Hospital Bereavement Services

. . . at the time of [an infant's] death, the role of the doctor is not obviated, but rather becomes infinitely more important.

LAWRENCE R. BERGER, M.D.

Although an increasing number of hospitals in Britain are adopting bereavement services to provide parents with practical and emotional help following a pregnancy loss, many hospitals still lack appropriate protocols.

Obstetricians, paediatricians, and hospital staff work under constant time pressures while juggling demands in both their training and their work. It is not surprising that they do not routinely learn the special skills required to help a family after a pregnancy loss has occurred, when their medical knowledge is no longer pertinent.

Yet the reasons for obstetrical, paediatric, and nursing departments to undertake such an investment in time and training are compelling. Helpful management of a pregnancy loss or newborn death has a profound and positive long-term effect on the family's emotional recovery and well-being. If you received skilled assistance in the hospital, you were better able to grieve and move past your untimely loss. Grieving helps to restore your healthy capacity for parenting a future child, which can otherwise be hindered. Trained hospital staff and physicians can help this healing process to begin.

Bereavement intervention skills give doctors and hospital staff a practical means of helping parents in distress, when they would otherwise feel ill-equipped to handle the emotional aspects of the loss. This training helps staff respect and manage their own sadness and anxiety as well.

Many nurses find that bereavement training improves their ability to help patients who suffered a pregnancy loss. One nurse explained that before she was trained, she had a typical staff response to a stillbirth she had witnessed. 'I was very upset,' she recalled. 'I was afraid that I couldn't help the patient because I was so emotional myself. I felt totally helpless.'

After attending a training programme she had learned to respect her own response to pregnancy loss:

I feel I can be more present and more emotionally available to the patient as a result. I know there are some things I can do for her, like show her the baby and let her talk and cry. These are small things, but they are important. I feel I have something to offer that will help.

When doctors and nurses begin to utilize bereavement interventions, they learn to tolerate patients' intense emotions and their own proximity to death. The lasting gratitude of bereaved parents usually convinces hospital staff that their training is both effective and worthwhile. 'The time and effort involved is less than might be expected,' explains one doctor. 'And in supporting families who are presented with one of life's greatest tragedies, no time and effort could be better spent.'

If you feel your needs were neglected during your hospital stay, you may wish to tell the hospital what could be done to help other parents in the future. You may get the best response through a patient representative, the social work department, the director of clinical services, or the hospital chaplain. One effective method is to write a letter to the person or department of your choice, with a copy to the hospital manager, requesting a follow-up meeting to discuss your experiences. The results of these efforts can be gratifying.

Laura felt the care surrounding her second-trimester pregnancy loss at a large hospital had been poorly handled, both medically and emotionally. Among other problems, she did not see or hold her baby girl when she was born, and she was initially told the hospital would not release the baby for burial because it weighed under five hundred grams. When her letter to the hospital's clerical director went unanswered, Laura asked to meet with the most senior midwife. The nurse listened to her story and verified it by checking the hospital records. She agreed Laura's experience had been unsatisfactory. The nursing supervisor then took up the matter with the head of obstetrics and the hospital management. Laura was pleased by how fruitful her efforts proved to be:

> Many changes occurred almost immediately. A camera was purchased, pictures and footprints are now kept on record, and a social worker is called in when a loss occurs. Parents are encouraged to see their babies, and private burial is offered as an option.

Not all hospitals respond so well to suggestions for improvement of their bereavement services, but when they do take patients' criticisms seriously, they allow bereaved parents to leave a legacy of compassion and help to others who suffer pregnancy losses after them.

If you act on your desire for change, you may discover your effort takes on special meaning, as it can become a way to honour your baby's memory. As Laura explained:

> My work on the hospital bereavement policies gave meaning to a life that never had a chance. It changed my grief and anger into positive action. It was a very, very good feeling to be productive in our baby's name.

What Can Help You Obtain Compassionate Medical Care

The emotional care and understanding your medical caregivers provided probably had a profound impact on you and your ability to grieve. If you were supported by staff trained in pregnancy loss and bereavement, your baby's importance and your sorrow were both recognized.

However, if the medical staff did not have specialized training, you probably did not receive consistently sensitive care following your loss, and you may suffer lasting regret. Weeks or months afterward, your mourning might be compounded by memories of upsetting incidents that occurred in your doctor's office or the hospital.

Some experiences you and your partner had in the hospital, and decisions you made about the baby, cannot be changed. You may, however, be able to repair some of the hurt afterward. Here are some suggestions:

- If you didn't request special care in the hospital, and now have regrets, try to forgive yourself, as you could not have known what you needed in the midst of your crisis. It is the hospital's responsibility to train staff who can provide this specialized care.
- If you feel your emotional care was mismanaged by your medical caregivers, it is important that you acknowledge and repair the hurt by talking about the incidents with someone you trust. If you continue to feel distressed, psychotherapy can help.
- If you experienced a late loss or newborn death, and the hospital failed to provide mementoes of your baby, check with the obstetric department. There is a possibility that footprints, a photograph, or other items may be on file and available to you.
- When you schedule your follow-up appointment with your doctor, ask for the first appointment of the morning or afternoon and remind

her to take you on time, so you can avoid waiting surrounded by pregnant women and new mothers.

- If you want to try to change the care provided by your doctor or your hospital, by all means write to each of them explaining your experience, what it meant to you, and what alternative care would have helped.

Bereavement Protocol

If you were dissatisfied with your hospital's bereavement services and want to recommend improvements to the hospital administrators, tell them a bereavement protocol would be helpful.

As a bereaved parent, you should have the opportunity:

- to contact your partner or support person
- to touch or hold your baby, before or after death; this may include you, your partner, your other children, and other relatives or close friends
- to be transferred from the maternity floor
- to receive pastoral care
- to name your baby
- to have a photograph of your baby to take home or for the hospital to keep on file
- to receive mementoes, including hospital birth certificate, footprints, baby's blanket, lock of hair, or identity bracelet
- to receive information on autopsy, burial, funeral, or memorial services
- to have the grieving process explained and to be provided with written information on bereavement
- to receive guidance on how to help your children at home cope with the loss
- to have the phone number of a staff person to call in case medical questions arise, or if you need emotional support or require referral information
- to receive follow-up appointments for medical tests and genetic counselling or to review laboratory and autopsy reports.

CHAPTER 10

· · · · · · · · · · · · · · · ·

FINDING SOLACE IN YOUR RELIGION

I wanted my religion to recognize that my stillborn daughter had existed, that she had been loved by us and by God.

CONNIE

When you suffer a pregnancy loss, you may turn toward and against your religion in the same moment. No matter when your loss occurred in the pregnancy, you deserve the comfort of knowning that your God has not forsaken you and that your baby has not gone from this world unnoticed or unblessed. Yet you may feel disturbed that the same God who is supposed to protect and console failed to safeguard your innocent child's life.

Few events shake religious faith more than losing a pregnancy. 'Experiences like ours make you doubt that things are well organized up there,' confessed Amelia after enduring two newborn deaths and a miscarriage. 'It makes you question the notion of any kind of cosmic justice.' Your grief may be so unmitigated that you begin to question everything about your faith.

You may find yourself bargaining with God after your loss, offering a new commitment to religion, to a more thoughtful life, to anything, if only your next pregnancy will produce a healthy baby. If additional losses or infertility occur, you may begin to feel truly abandoned by your God.

If you turn to a well-trained and compassionate member of the clergy for counsel, you will probably find an appropriate way to release your doubts and anger. Once you give expression to your sorrow in a spiritually meaningful way, you may once again find solace in your religion. If, however, the member of the clergy you turn to for help does not comfort you or denies you ritual acknowledgment of your grief, your frustration and anger toward your religion – and even God – can become overpowering.

Birth and death remain the ultimate mysteries of life, and the death of a baby during or shortly after pregnancy is especially troubling. People, including the clergy, are so unsettled by pregnancy loss and infant death that they tend to offer platitudes such as 'It was God's will' or 'It happened for the best.' As one father argued, 'If things always happened for the best there would be no pregnancy loss in the world to begin with.'

The profound period of doubt you may be experiencing after your loss does not necessarily mark the end of your faith. 'It may even be a new beginning,' maintains Matthew Ripley-Moffitt, a Protestant minister. 'Your crisis may cause you to go through a transition of faith development, rather than destruction.'

For some parents, the trial of sorrow deepens their spiritual life and enriches their relationships with family, friends, and congregants at their house of worship. These parents gain a new respect for the preciousness of life, which they may interpret as a parting gift from their baby or a lesson taught by God.

If you are struggling to find solace in your religion, do not be surprised, however, if your faith is shaken to the core. There is still hope for you to achieve the consolation you need – and deserve.

When Your Loss Feels Like Retribution

*L*ike many parents, you probably wonder why this misfortune befell you and your baby. Up until this point, your life may have seemed like a series of challenges followed by rewards for each success. So when you are faced with the grief of losing a pregnancy or an innocent baby, the need to find a reason, any reason, is a natural attempt to grasp the ungraspable. Since most major religions espouse concepts of sin and retribution, you may begin to feel a strong dose of anger and guilt mixed in with your sorrow. 'If bad things only happen to bad people,' one woman wondered, 'what did I do to deserve this punishment? And my child was so innocent. How could God have done this to my baby?'

You may feel guilty for not having planned the pregnancy you lost, for aborting a previous pregnancy, or for feeling ambivalent about becoming a parent. Martha found it particularly difficult to be Catholic and single when she suffered her first-trimester miscarriage. 'A lot of the nurses in the hospital were catholics too and I felt they were judging me,' she admitted. 'Even when I asked to speak to my own priest, I felt more guilty than comforted. I felt I was suffering from having sinned rather than from having been the victim of a loss.' It is no wonder that you may find yourself doubting your faith. 'If my religion can't comfort me at a time like this,' professed one mother, 'what good is it?'

When You Turn to the Clergy

Parents ask me, 'How can I believe in God when my baby dies?' And priests in turn must ask themselves the question, 'How do I affirm life when its greatest symbol, a little baby, is taken away?'

THE REVEREND DR VIENNA COBB ANDERSON, Episcopal priest

Your clergyperson's response to your sorrow can greatly affect the degree of solace you obtain from your faith. If your rabbi, priest, or minister listens to your concerns and offers relevant rituals, even your negative emotions, such as anger or guilt, can be released, allowing healthy grieving to begin. On the other hand, if the cleric you turn to has not been trained in bereavement counselling and offers only platitudes or denies you meaningful ceremonies, your anger may be unleashed at your religion and at God.

When the Clergy Console You

When sensitive pastoral care is offered, you can be truly consoled by your faith. Members of the clergy who show their human side, who are able to grieve with your family, who listen more than they speak, and who do not dismiss your desire for ritual can be enormously effective.

Amelia's minister was willing to reach out to her and her husband throughout their difficult reproductive history, offering prayers, baptism, and a memorial service for each loss. 'But what I remember most about my minister, what affected me the most,' explained Amelia, 'was that at our first baby's memorial service he was constantly wiping his eyes and blowing his nose. He was so human.'

There are sensitive members of the clergy and funeral directors who offer comforting rituals for pregnancy loss. If you feel the clergyperson you have contacted is too constrained by tradition, try to find another person whose training and creativity are more appealing to you. The hospital social worker or chaplain may be able to help.

Connie called her parish priest after her stillbirth because she wanted a ceremony but didn't know what would be appropriate. He told her that the Catholic Church felt a stillborn baby's soul went straight to heaven and that it wasn't necessary to name her baby or have a burial service for her.

Connie was not satisfied with her priest's response, so she called the hospital and asked to speak with their Catholic priest, even though she had already been discharged. He helped her make arrangements with a compassionate funeral director so her daughter could have the right burial – the kind she and her husband wanted. 'The hospital chaplain also gave me a candle to light at home,' recalled Connie, 'a small gesture, but one that meant a great deal to me because it was so tangible.'

If the member of the clergy you turn to for help comforts you, writing a note of thanks can be a wonderful gesture. Often the clergy themselves are not certain if they have said or done the right thing. Having the expressed gratitude of a parent can help them realize that their long hours and sincere attempts to serve God and humanity are worthwhile.

When Religion May Disappoint You

You may feel disheartened if your desire for religious solace is thwarted after your loss. This could be the first time you have turned to the clergy for guidance, and you may expect them to know just how to help you.

Spiritual leaders have to wrestle with theology, questions of faith, and their congregants' grief, all while considering their own sadness and mortality. Like other people, members of the clergy often feel especially helpless when trying to explain infant death or pregnancy loss.

Some priests, ministers, and rabbis compound the situation by setting themselves above grief and tears, either as an example of fortitude or for self-protection. A greater problem is that most members of the clergy receive little training in bereavement counselling during their formal education. Hospital chaplains are the most likely to have bereavement training, but their exposure to pregnancy loss and infant death may still be minimal. This lack of preparation can leave members of the clergy so out of touch with the needs of bereaved parents that they may make errors of judgment and taste.

Adam was dismayed when a member of the clergy, whom he had driven to his baby's grave site for a service, brought up the payment of his fee on the way home. Adam was grateful for the tenderness the pastor had put into the brief service, so he was astonished by the sudden discussion of remuneration. 'I felt he should have mentioned his fee during our initial conversation when we planned the service,' admitted Adam. 'It left us with an unhappy feeling about him and our religion.'

If you are planning a service for your baby, try to keep several issues in mind. Be sure the clergyperson conducting the ritual knows your infant's name, because having it omitted or mispronounced can make you feel as if your child was not cherished. You may want to inquire if your priest, minister, or rabbi maintains a calendar system to keep track of appropriate anniversaries, so that you will be contacted a year later, when you might be feeling particularly sad. If your cleric does not have a system, you may want to let her know you would appreciate a follow-up call. This is one way you can improve upon your clergyperson's understanding of pregnancy loss; at the same time, you may leave a legacy of better pastoral care in your congregation.

If you suffered a midterm or late loss, you may have contacted a funeral director, whose training and compassion are important when you are so vulnerable.

Irene was equally disturbed when immediately after the conclusion of the grave site ceremony for her stillborn daughter, she heard the sound of a loud motor revving and turned to see a digger lumbering over to fill her baby's grave. 'It was rude,' Irene complained. 'They should have waited a while, at least until the family had left.'

If you are a member of a denomination that encourages large families, you may begin to feel as if you had failed not only yourself but also your faith by experiencing a pregnancy loss. After several miscarriages, Julia found it uncomfortable to go to church every Sunday and be surrounded by the many pregnant women and large families in her congregation. She became additionally upset when one pregnant member of the congregation informed her, 'When God wants you to have a baby, you'll have a baby.' Julia felt differently. 'Maybe God has provided doctors with the knowledge to help me achieve a family,' she surmised. 'Isn't that a gift from God, too? I couldn't believe that God was failing me any more than I was failing God.'

If you receive thoughtless treatment from a member of the clergy, a funeral director, cemetery staff, or someone in your congregation, try to vent your anger by expressing your displeasure. If you do not want to bring up your concerns in person, consider writing a letter. Even professionals may not realize how offensive their shortcomings are unless bereaved parents take the time to educate them. Remember, however, that it is equally important to write a letter if you have received compassionate care.

The Relevance of Rituals

Rituals can help you to say goodbye to your baby and begin a healthy grieving response; they also serve as a signal to the larger community that you deserve special attention and care following your loss.

Like many parents, this may be the first time you have had to say goodbye to a loved one or make burial arrangements. You may have no idea what is considered correct or suitable, and you may be unprepared for the impact these decisions have on you and your partner. Irene remembered the difficulty she and her husband had deciding where their stillborn daughter should be buried. 'We had to discuss our own mortality,' she recalled, 'and how and where we wanted to be buried ourselves.'

The clergy may inadvertently confuse you by not giving you clear information about your options, suggesting that you do 'whatever you want' when you have no idea what you want. Some parents find these concerns so painful that they shy away from planning a ritual goodbye for their baby. They hope their sorrow will fade with time if they avoid a ceremony.

Although it is difficult for many parents to think about expressing their grief in front of others, even loved ones, rituals provide a cathartic moment to release the pain, to acknowledge the loss, and to start to grieve. Amelia and her husband knew they wanted a memorial service in the hospital where their premature baby had lived her short life:

> It seems to me that by acknowledging our baby's death with a ritual, we were acknowledging that our baby lived and that she had made a difference in a lot of people's lives, even though hers was so short. If we hadn't done something, it would have been like sweeping her ashes out into the street.

For Laura, planning a ritual goodbye for her baby who had not survived a premature delivery became a way of turning an unbearable shock into a comprehensible sorrow. Although her rabbi tried to dissuade her from attending the funeral, Laura believed that being there was the only way the loss could ever become real to her. 'I instinctively knew I needed to go to the funeral,' she admitted. 'It was the only normal thing that happened through the whole ordeal.'

Sometimes the mother can't attend a planned ritual because she is still in hospital and the funeral can't be postponed. If this happens, keep the burial as scheduled but arrange a memorial service later, when the mother can attend. Another solution is to make a video- or audiotape of the service so she has a record of the ceremony to keep. It is also helpful if the hospitalized mother is allowed to plan as much of the ceremony as possible and if a close relative, friend, or member of the clergy stays with her during the service.

Many hospitals offer an ecumenical memorial service for all pregnancy losses and infant deaths once a year, usually around Christmas. Participating in this annual ritual can be comforting to parents who have been unable to attend the burial of their baby or who had a first-trimester loss.

If cremation is an option, and none of these other alternatives is available, you might give it consideration. Ashes can be interred at any point following the loss, so cremation may be a sensitive, accommodating solution.

Naming Your Baby

The moment we knew it was a daughter we named her Melanie, and she has been Melanie ever since. By naming her, I have acknowledged that she was very real to me, and I can refer to her in a very real way. And it is a name I can never use again. I had a daughter named Melanie.

RUTH

Few rituals give more concreteness to a loss than naming the child. And few rites could be more simple. Although many parents may not wish to acknowledge an early loss in this way, some do, and they should be allowed this comfort. Most members of the clergy encourage naming infants born of later losses as a way of affirming the unique identity of the baby and the baby's place in the family.

Naming your baby allows you to refer to your child personally with love and honour, and it helps the grieving process by lending reality to both the baby and your loss. 'It seems to me the ultimate non-identity is to refer to a baby as "it,"' said Amelia, who named both of her premature babies who died shortly after birth. 'It would have been hard always to refer to John, for example, only as "the boy baby who died."'

Some parents are afraid they'll never find another name they love, so they 'save' the name and give the child one they don't like as much. However, parents who give their deceased baby the name they had already chosen are usually glad to have done so and find that naming subsequent children is not the problem they had anticipated. As one mother who had suffered two losses revealed, 'After we named both babies, we wondered if there would be a name left we liked. But as soon as we named the next baby, who lived, we loved that name, too.'

The issue becomes more complicated if religious tradition and family expectations maintain that children should be named for a beloved relative, living or dead. Couples may feel they are not providing the proper honour in bestowing the name on a child who has already died or has no hope of living. Lisa, whose Jewish tradition of naming babies after a deceased relative meant a great deal to her, explained her thoughts when her baby was born to live only a few hours:

> We had picked out names after our grandparents. When we knew she was not expected to live, I didn't want to use the names. We started thinking that she should be named after both of us, her parents, because she was such a part of us. That's not the Jewish tradition, but it was important to us. So we gave her two names, each one starting with our own first initials.

If you had decided not to name your child and now have regrets, it is a decision you can change at a later time.

Burying or Cremating Your Baby

Formal burial or cremation is a legal requirement for all 24-week babies who are stillborn or who die after birth and is optional for babies who die before this legal age of viability. Although for some faiths, it is important that the funeral should take place as soon as possible, in general, there is no need to make decisions about your baby's funeral in a hurry. The hospital should reassure you that your baby's body can be kept safely until you have made up your mind how best to honour your baby. At a time when you were planning your baby's future, it is so shocking to have to make arrangements for a funeral. You may feel that you cannot or don't want to do this yourselves and may prefer that the hospital take care of it. All hospitals will arrange and pay for a basic funeral for your baby if born after 24 weeks and some will provide a funeral for babies born before 24 weeks. When making your decision, it helps to have details about which cemetery or crematorium is used or other memorials the hospital might suggest for your baby. Although hospitals will usually encourage the parents to take part in planning and attending the funeral, parents may still loose control over what happens to their baby. This may be a source of regret later, even for those parents who couldn't bear to be involved at the time.

If you want to organize the funeral, the first step is to contact a funeral director. Hospitals will usually give you a list of local funeral directors, although you are not obliged to follow their recommendations. You can discuss costs in advance and it is possible to have a simple funeral which costs very little. It is not difficult to organize a funeral, requiring only one or two calls, or visits. Sometimes a friend or relative can do this for you.

When you are deciding whether to have your baby's body buried or cremated, it helps to have further information about each of these choices. Sometimes there are local regulations which may affect your options.

If a baby is cremated, it is important to know that there may be no ashes. This is because the soft bones of very small babies are usually destroyed by the high temperatures used in cremation. However, some crematoria can provide ashes. Parents may be able to erect a small plaque in the grounds of the crematorium. If there are ashes, parents may prefer to scatter them in a place with special meaning, or bury them in an urn in a crematorium or churchyard that is nearer to their home.

If you are organizing a funeral yourselves, you will probably have to pay for a grave, which is likely to be the most expensive part of the funeral. If the hospital arranges the burial, it is usually in a grave with other babies. You may find it comforting to know that your baby will not be alone.

Coffins for babies are very small and are usually made from a white polyurethane material which some parents dislike. Other types of coffins are available.

You may find it comforting to choose something special for your baby to wear or to select objects to be placed in the coffin with her. Making these small but important arrangements may provide a connection with your baby that you need. 'I put in a couple of toys, a blanket and little socks, ruffled socks', recalled Irene about the day before her stillborn daughter's burial. 'It was so hard buying them, but it meant a lot to my husband and me to have those things with her.'

Funeral director, Ronald Troyer suggests that bereaved parents plan a meal or other informal gathering following any burial or cremation to give family and friends the chance to share in the open recognition of the couples' grief. He feels that giving the parents the opportunity to bond with their family and friends can help in reducing the conspiracy of silence parents often feel at future family and social gatherings.

If the thought of a funeral service is too painful, you may find a simple memorial service to be a less distressing way for you and your family to say goodbye to your baby.

When Ritual Is Denied

If you feel you need a traditional ritual in recognition of your sorrow, it is very upsetting to have a member of the clergy try to dissuade you from performing a rite you believe will be comforting. When the clergy are not well trained in these issues, or when they are overwhelmed by their own feelings of sorrow and helplessness, they tend to lead bereaved parents away from rituals. They may encourage you to get on with your life, to plan another pregnancy and not use ritual as a means of expressing your grief. Although this advice comes from good intentions, it couldn't be more misguided.

Members of the clergy may deny grieving parents rites because of theological constraints or confusion over the appropriateness of employing certain standard rituals for the death of a baby. Catholic priests and Protestant ministers may refuse to baptize a stillborn baby, since baptism is a sacrament reserved only for the living. The Jewish tradition of sitting shiva, in which mourners receive visitors at home for seven days, is not encouraged. Jewish parents also may be dissuaded from having a funeral service for a baby who did not live the requisite thirty-day period beyond birth established by Jewish law, although burial is required.

Adele asked to see a rabbi after her premature daughter died shortly after delivery at twenty-one weeks. She wasn't sure what she wanted to do or what was even proper, but Adele knew she didn't want her baby simply disposed of by the hospital without some religious ritual:

> I wanted to know if there was any special prayer we could say. The rabbi said there wasn't any. He also tried to talk us out of a funeral, saying it wasn't necessary and would be too expensive. I got the feeling he says this to all women, but he didn't realize how much I had committed to the pregnancy and what I had been through.

Laura found that the absence of religious ritual for her premature baby made it more difficult for other people, especially those in her congregation, to cope with the situation. Even though she eventually convinced her rabbi that she needed to have a funeral, the ceremony included only the immediate family:

> If we had been allowed to have a ritual recognized by the community,

it would have given others a way to acknowledge our grief. Since we couldn't sit shiva, there was no way for people to recognize and share our grief, so they said nothing, which was much worse.

I would have felt my pain and attachment to this baby had been validated if there had been a prescribed way for people to respond to us. Without rituals, I felt embarrassed and ashamed, as if I had done something wrong because my baby had died.

If you or the member of the clergy you have turned to for help doubt that religious rituals are meaningful and important, their value becomes clear in its absence. Omission of rituals can be an attempt to erase the painful reality of your loss. With time, you may realize these efforts were futile, and you might even feel negligent toward your child for not having provided a ritual. If this is your situation, you can name your baby or hold a memorial service at a later date to help bring a feeling of closure to your grief.

The Need for Special Rituals

If you have decided that traditional rituals are not a suitable way to commemorate your loss, you may still feel the need to have some observance that is personal and meaningful. You may find solace in honouring your child's birth date or due date, perhaps by reading aloud a letter or poem you have written to your baby, as well as setting aside time just to recall the brief moments you shared, even if they existed only during your pregnancy.

Planting a tree or perennial shrub in honour of your baby may provide the sense of ritual and symbolism you need. A member of the clergy could participate, and this could be another opportunity to read prayers, a poem, or a letter you have written to your baby. You might want to honour your baby by committing yourself to a meaningful volunteer project or by making a charitable donation in the baby's name. Some hospitals have books they will inscribe with your baby's name if you choose to make a donation. You may want to mark the baby's death and birth by visiting the hospital and looking at the book.

The personal ritual you create might change over time once your loss is more integrated into your life. After Wendy buried two newborn babies, she placed flowers on their graves every week. Later, she began to feel she had gone past the need to make the weekly trip but still wanted to commemorate her children in a tangible way, to show that they were with her in spirit. So each Monday she has fresh flowers delivered to her office. 'I think of the flowers as a gift from my children,' she claims. 'It helps me to look at my flowers every day and for people at work to see them, too. It's as if my children are still spreading joy.' See Appendix B, on rituals, for additional suggestions.

Rituals for Early Losses

All but one of my losses were so early we didn't even consider rituals. But we regret not doing something more. We didn't put the emotional energy into grieving that we should have.

VERA

If you suffered an early loss and feel the need for a ritual, do not hesitate to speak to the hospital chaplain or the head of your own congregation. Because you will have nothing more than blood or 'fetal tissue,' services such as funerals and burials are often discouraged by the clergy as being too expensive and unwarranted, but this does not mean your loss should go unacknowledged or your baby unblessed.

Ellen had experienced several first-trimester miscarriages and only gradually realized her need for ritual was growing with each loss. By the time she suffered her fifth miscarriage, she felt compelled to acknowledge her sorrow in some religious way. As she sat bleeding and cramping in a hospital emergency room, Ellen was startled when a hospital volunteer came up to her and asked if she could bring her anything:

> It just sort of popped out of me, without much forethought, that I wanted to speak with a hospital chaplain, who arrived a few minutes later. He was a kind, soft-spoken priest who asked what he could do for me. I told him I wanted a prayer for the baby who had died inside of me. He stood quietly by my chair and said a gentle, simple prayer that acknowledged my love for my baby, no matter how small it was. Few religious services in my life have touched me more deeply.

If you feel the need to commemorate your early loss, please read the prayers, poems, and rituals in Appendix B, and contact a member of the clergy if you wish to express your grief in a more formal way.

Rituals for Ending an Impaired Pregnancy

*F*ew situations present a more searing theological problem than abortion. Indeed, as entire populations struggle with this issue, people from all walks of life, including lawmakers, politicians, and doctors, as well as members of the clergy, are drawn into the conflagration. But as long as antenatal testing exists and the struggle is borne privately in the hearts of bereaved parents and their physicians, religious leaders must accept that mothers and fathers who are ending their pregnancies need and deserve the comfort of their faith.

This does not pose much of a problem for liberal Protestant or Jewish denominations, but the Catholic Church, Orthodox Judaism, and fundamentalist Christian sects are generally opposed to any form of abortion. However, people of these faiths should still be entitled to spiritual help and rituals to assuage their grief when they decide to end their pregnancies. 'So many people feel guilty about the decision, they don't feel they deserve to be sad,' explains Catherine Garlid, a Protestant hospital chaplain. 'But that can really complicate the grieving process. It is just as crucial that these parents get support, help, and comfort, too.'

If you are one such bereaved parent, you have experienced a real and painful loss rendered more agonizing by the issue of choice. You need to mourn, and if this includes seeking out the comfort of your religion, you should be able to find solace within your faith. You should be allowed to bury or cremate your baby, to have a memorial service, funeral, or anything else you need to acknowledge your sorrow.

Even the more conservative lines are softening somewhat on this issue. One Orthodox rabbi explained that although his denomination rejects the idea of abortion, 'In no way is a baby to be rejected or despised.' He insists that burial of an Orthodox baby under these circumstances is still possible and that no sanctions are implemented against the parents for making the choice to abort.

Devout Catholics and fundamentalist Christians may have the most difficulty, since any abortion is forbidden by their religion. Many of them simply forgo antenatal testing as a result. However, certain routine antenatal examinations can indicate defects that are incompatible with life. If these parents wish to abort a pregnancy, they should be encouraged to seek out private counselling with a compassionate priest or minister.

If you cannot find a helpful member of the clergy who understands your need for religious acknowledgment of your loss, ask a hospital social worker for guidance. She should be able to put you in touch with an understanding clergyperson, perhaps one of the hospital chaplains.

Your Return to Faith

*E*ven if you have become a lapsed practitioner of your religion, you may turn to old beliefs for comfort in the desolation of losing your baby. Your experience may deepen your faith and commitment to God. For some parents, the joy of a subsequent baby gives them a renewed trust in their religion. For others, the loss itself becomes the key to a restoration of faith.

Wendy struggled with her faith when she lost two newborn babies. With the first loss, she was overwhelmed by guilt that she had done something wrong, and she blamed God for punishing her. After her second loss, her attitude shifted and she began to believe that she could try to learn something from her sorrow instead:

> Little by little I am returning to my faith. I want to have faith in something. I want to belive in something again. This has really shattered my life. I can't believe this is the only life my children have had. I want to believe my children are in a better place.

Even with a renewal of faith, religious doubts can continue to plague you. But doubts can strengthen faith, just as questions advance learning. You may find the experience of grappling with the issues – even if they sometimes remain unresolved – has a positive effect on your life. Ellen recalled talking to a local priest when she was a teenager, a conversation that had remained forgotten for years until after she had endured several miscarriages:

> He said the point of religion was not to explain away bad things but to equip us to handle them. So what it came down to for me was not what all my pregnancy losses meant in a religious sense, because ultimately I don't think they happened for any real purpose. There was no Divine Plan, no Ultimate Test.
>
> But what *I* made of the losses, how they affected my life, that was the real test of my faith. Could I do some good as a result of my sorrow? Would I be able to overcome my bitterness and still love life? That was the challenge – and the final comfort I'll probably spend the rest of my life striving for. God was within me with the babies I lost, but I am the

only one who can build into my life a memorial to the children I will never see grow up.

What Can Help You Find Solace In Your Religion

When you lose a baby during or shortly after pregnancy, your faith may be badly shaken. You may doubt your belief in an orderly universe overseen by a loving, compassionate God. When members of the clergy fail to offer you the words and rituals you need to acknowledge your sorrow and express your grief, you may become even more disillusioned with your religion.

But there are many appropriate ways to seek the solace you yearn for, even if you feel momentarily abandoned by your congregation, your pastor, or your faith. Here are some suggestions that might help you to find the comfort within your religion that you deserve:

- If you turn to a member of the clergy who does not offer what you need, consider looking further. There are compassionate clerics and funeral directors who can guide you toward the rituals and comforts for which you yearn. Consider contacting the social worker or chaplain at the hospital where your loss occurred.
- If you do not need a public acknowledgment of your loss in which you participate, think about asking a member of the clergy to offer a prayer on your behalf as part of a regular religious service or during their private devotions.
- Consider naming your child to give the baby an identity, so you can refer to your infant with the specific warmth and affection parents reserve for their children.
- If you decide to bury your child, contemplate buying a little outfit for him to wear or toys to be placed in the coffin or grave.
- If the mother cannot attend the funeral or burial service for medical reasons, try to postpone it until she is able to attend. If this is impossible, schedule a memorial service after she has recuperated, or tape the burial for her. Be sure she has someone to stay with her during the ceremony if she cannot attend.
- Consider composing poems or prayers to your baby that can be read aloud at a funeral or memorial service. You may want to plant a tree

or a perennial flower in honour of your baby that you can watch grow over the years, or make a charitable donation to honour your baby's memory.

- If you receive thoughtless care by a member of the clergy or someone else you feel should have known better, think about writing to the person who offended you. Try to remember what a kindness it is also to write a note of thanks when your care has been suitable and comforting.
- Endeavour to accept that bad things sometimes happen for no reason at all and that the only meaning you can give your tragic loss is how you cope with it and how you integrate it into your life.

THE RESPONSE OF YOUR FAMILY AND FRIENDS

During your first moments of sorrow, compassionate friends and relatives may have comforted you, listening to your story and letting you cry. But even those who love you may not understand the depth of your grief or the length of time it might take you to feel better. Pregnancy loss remains a taboo subject in our society, so even the most caring relatives and friends may not know how to help you cope with your sorrow – while you feel equally ill-equipped to guide them.

In the coming days and weeks, you and your partner must justify your absence from work and inform family and friends whom you do not see regularly that you lost the baby. Explaining your loss to this wider circle can leave you feeling more drained and angry than supported, especially if people's responses seem clumsy or inappropriate.

This chapter can help you secure the comfort you need from others and enable you to deal with your disappointment when you do not get the support you deserve. You might want to encourage family and friends to read this section of the book, especially if they would like to help you through this difficult time but aren't sure of the best approach.

Telling People About Your Loss

Breaking the news of your pregnancy loss to others can be a heartbreaking and overwhelming task. Your own immediate reactions of shock and dismay may turn to a sense of embarrassment and failure as you are forced to tell your story over and over again. Whether you are informing loved ones or acquaintances about your loss, you must explain your tragedy, often exposing your own raw emotions.

Informing Close Family and Friends

As much as you need to reach out to loved ones after your loss, you may feel you are intruding on their lives by sharing such sad news. If your family recently enjoyed a happy occasion, such as a wedding, your announcement can seem to cover their high spirits with a shroud of gloom. On the other hand, if they have experienced recent sorrows, you may feel you are only augmenting their sadness. 'I don't like calling people with bad news,' said Linda as she remembered the first few weeks following the death of her newborn baby, 'so I waited for them to call me.'

Once you feel ready to talk about your loss, you need willing listeners who can make you feel loved and valued. Your own parents may be the first people you call, but their ability to respond helpfully can depend on the quality of your relationship with them.

Julia phoned her mother immediately after she had suffered her second miscarriage:

> She cried as soon as I told her. If I needed her to go anywhere or do anything, she was there for me. She didn't reflect everything back on herself. She just listened to me and dealt with my emotions. My feelings were her concern.

Your parents may be able to put you first and show their support by being with you or offering practical help, such as putting away baby things or taking care of your other children. But pregnancy loss is a misfortune for grandparents as well. They may be preoccupied by their own sorrow or worried about the mother's physical health. As a result, they may give unwanted advice instead of expressing pure love and concern.

Simple, comforting words are often more appreciated than well-meaning advice. One woman remembered how different each of her parent's remarks had been when she told them about her fourth miscarriage and D&C:

> My mother openly asked me why I kept going through pregnancies and miscarriages, and she urged me to stop doing this to my body. But my father just told me how much he loved me and that he would support me no matter what I decided to do. Of the two, my father was far more comforting.

For a more detailed discussion of the impact pregnancy loss has on grandparents, please read Chapter 13, 'For Bereaved Grandparents.'

Close friends pose particular problems. Some may not realize how upset you are and avoid the subject of the loss or utter thoughtless remarks, a topic that is discussed later in this chapter. Others may truly help, offering to bring over a meal or make necessary phone calls. Sometimes simple expressions of genuine sympathy are meaningful. 'When I told one of my best friends about my miscarriage,' recalled Ellen, 'her eyes immediately filled with tears. She didn't say much, but she conveyed her own sorrow and disappointment, which meant so much to me.'

Telling Your Wider Social Circle

Once you have told your immediate family members and friends about your loss, you face informing colleagues and other acquaintances. Some parents find they accept their loss a little more each time they tell another person. But this process can be extremely difficult as you listen to people's reactions, perhaps attempting to comfort them while still immersed in your own sadness. Each person you tell may want to talk about the loss at length, compelling you to repeat your story when you already feel depressed and overburdened.

You should feel free to ask close friends and family to call other people, so you will not be overwhelmed by this unhappy task. You can also look for a more protected way to tell others about your loss. In America several charities publish cards especially designed for this situation. In gentle, appealing phrases the cards express the parents' sorrow and suggest how the recipient can offer support. They also include a place to record the baby's name, birth date, and weight. One bereaved mother sent a card issued by one of those charities which read:

> Acknowledgment of our child's short life may be upsetting to you. You may think the less said the better. Until now we did now know how important it would be for us to tell you of our little baby, even though our baby died. You can help us through this difficult time by letting us talk about our sorrow when we feel the need, allowing us to cry when we want and not pretending that everything is okay . . . when it's not. It will take time, but with your support we will make it.

– You could consider using these words on your own card.

Paul, whose baby daughter was stillborn, was most comfortable writing personal notes to people outside his immediate friends and family:

> I picked a card with a stark photograph of a bleak landscape, an overcast day with a lone tree clinging to the side of a mountain. I

wrote a note explaining what had happened, and I heard back from people, which was wonderful. Most of them wrote to me, which was easier than handling all those phone calls.

Comments from well-meaning people who knew about the pregnancy but were not aware of the loss can be especially difficult. It is important to keep in mind that these people are only showing interest and support by asking about your pregnancy. They do not intend to hurt you with their questions, as painful or awkward as they may seem. You cannot avoid embarrassing them a little by telling the truth, but you can ease the situation by making your response as straightforward as possible. Planning and practising what to say beforehand can help you find comfortable phrases that discourage unwanted questions.

Two months after she lost her full-term son to congenital abnormalities, Linda ran into a woman she knew slightly who commented on the fact that she was no longer pregnant and asked if she had a boy or a girl. Linda had thought carefully about how she would handle this predicament, so she was prepared with a response:

> I tried to use the gentlest language possible in these situations, not mentioning death or the baby's abnormalities. I just said: 'I had a son, but he didn't make it.' She got the message that I didn't want to say any more than that.

Telling acquaintances about your loss may be harder than telling family and friends. The people you and your partner feel closest to are probably more comfortable seeing you cry and sharing their own grief without becoming embarrassed. You might feel awkward breaking down in front of people you don't know well, or annoyed by having to comfort them when they become upset about your news. Amelia found herself in this situation when she attended the first performance in a series of plays following the death of her premature baby. She dreaded facing the couple who had sat next to her and her husband for the entire series:

> They weren't close friends, but they were aware of our baby's illness and I knew they would ask about her. I knew I was going to have to tell them, but it seemed so unfair to say 'She died' right before the lights went out and the curtain went up. What would they be able to say to us at intermission? I couldn't avoid making them uncomfortable no matter how or when I chose to tell them.

Try to be realistically prepared for the awkwardness of these situations when you know in advance they might occur. Opening with something like 'I know this will come as a shock' or 'I have sad news to tell you' gives people a little time to brace themselves for their own reactions. It is inevitable that they will still feel uncomfortable or upset, but try not to take on the burden of their feelings in addition to your own suffering.

Mothers can find it especially helpful to alert colleagues first before returning to work full-time, perhaps telephoning and asking a supervisor to inform the rest of the office. Molly, who worked in a large advertising agency, was relieved to discover that her boss had sent out a letter to all of their clients after her baby was stillborn. 'I actually appreciated it very much,' she recalled. 'Not only was I spared having to tell the news myself, I got so many letters of condolence in return. People really poured their hearts out to me in those letters.'

Arranging lunch with colleagues before returning to work full-time can also make your transitions easier. It gives your colleagues the chance to ask the usual questions and enables you to answer without having to turn immediately back to your desk and work responsibilities.

Even if you and your partner take these precautions, be prepared for some slipups. If this happens, try to explain your story in terms that are easy for you to handle. This will keep you from having an overly emotional response at an awkward time.

Linda had alerted most of her colleagues about her newborn son's death, but word had not spread throughout her company by the time she returned to work:

> When one of the managers in another department saw me, she exclaimed, 'Oh, you're back so soon! How's everything going? What did you have?' I pulled her into an empty office and told her in scientific terms what had happened. If I had told her more of the emotional elements, I would have broken down, and I didn't want to.

If you are a single woman, you may have additional concerns about announcing your loss to this wider social circle, even if you had planned your pregnancy. The awkward silence or embarrassment of colleagues and managers can make you feel an unspoken disapproval of your pregnancy instead of sympathy for your loss. If you need additional sources of comfort, a psychotherapist or a group like SANDS should be able to provide you with the consolation you deserve without submitting you to needless judgment.

Special Circumstances

*I*f your baby suffered from birth defects, you probably want to avoid inappropriate remarks or prying questions from even close friends and family, as well as colleagues and acquaintances. You may find it helpful to decide how much you want to reveal to each person on an individual basis.

Adam, whose baby had a fatal congenital disorder and lived only a few hours after birth, felt this approach eased the strain of each encounter:

> We didn't know how necessary it was to tell all the details about the loss to people, especially to those who didn't know us well, but you do need to express the truth at times. We decided differently with each person we told.

If your loss included having labour induced, you may be exposed to unintentionally hurtful remarks as well. Family and friends may refer to the 'abortion' rather than the loss, completely negating your experience of losing a wanted baby.

Paula had leaked so much amniotic fluid during her fifth month that her doctors urged her to abandon the pregnancy by inducing labour. She was upset when she returned to work to find people saying how sorry they were that she had to have an abortion rather than expressing their sadness over her loss. 'After that,' admitted Paula, 'I just told people I leaked fluid and lost the baby, without even mentioning inducement.'

If your loss involved induction of labour or your baby had severe birth defects, think about the explanations you want to give each person individually. Try to convey what the loss meant to you so that others will be more able to respond helpfully and compassionately.

Finding the Support You Need

You can't expect people who have not gone through a pregnancy loss to understand what it is all about.

ERIC

Shortly after your loss, you may begin to feel bereft of support and solace not only from friends and family but also from the entire community. Standard religious customs and ceremonies are often not available to bereaved parents following pregnancy loss and newborn death, a topic that is explored more fully in Chapter 10, 'Finding Solace in Your Religion.' You may find this lack of support and comfort from society upsetting, as if the world had forgotten how to reach out to you in your grief, making your loss a truly unacknowledged sorrow.

If friends and family seem unsure of what to say or do, it is probably because they have not experienced a similar tragedy. People seem to have lost a common thread of custom, as well as a willingness to share misfortunes with each other. The fact that pregnancy loss can be a hidden, almost taboo subject is also partly to blame. Even family members who suffered a loss may have kept it secret until you told them about yours.

Social customs surrounding death used to be very important. The clothing people wore, the sprig of flowers or the purple wreath on the door enabled everyone in the community to know that a family was in need and required special attention and care. People knew about the death and cooked meals, or called and just came by.

We've lost that important sense of community around death, especially that of an unborn or newborn child and by relying on the telephone to spread the news, people end up feeling even more removed from the event:

As one minister said:

> So often I hear members of my congregation say they didn't bother to visit people in mourning because they would probably cry and upset everybody, without realizing that this is exactly what should happen, that people are more upset if they *don't* see their friends and relatives crying with them.
>
> Most of us feel we have to keep life nice. We are afraid of pain and vulnerability and the tenuousness of life. And nothing seems to leave us feeling more vulnerable or tenuous than the death of an innocent baby.

When people overcome these obstacles and reach out to you, it can be especially meaningful and helpful. Even if your friends and family have never shared a similar sorrow, they can help you by offering to put away baby items or calling a store to cancel an order for baby equipment. One grieving mother remembered a friend who brought a meal for her and her husband while she was recuperating from an early miscarriage:

> We weren't up to going out yet and we hated the idea of cooking for ourselves, so it was a wonderful gesture. She even stayed to clean up afterwards in the kitchen. I know she could never know exactly how I

felt, because she had never suffered a loss herself, but what she did was so loving and thoughtful.

Handling Thoughtless Remarks

You may feel exhausted and frustrated by the effort to reach out to people after your pregnancy loss, especially when you are still immersed in your own grief. One of the greatest disappointments comes when friends and family you expected to be the first to offer comfort fail to supply the solace you need.

Family members and close friends usually want to be supportive, but sometimes their attempts to offer consolation backfire miserably. When people don't know what to say they may blurt out the most preposterous statements. However well-meaning the intention, comments such as 'It happened for the best' or 'You can always have another baby' do not acknowledge the sorrow or the loss you feel.

People often overlook the simplest statement when trying to say something comforting. Even conveying the thought 'I don't know what to say' acknowledges your sorrow and the awkwardness many people feel at such a time, without denying you some solace.

When Eve returned to work after an early miscarriage and a colleague said to her, 'I'm so sorry, I know how much you wanted that baby,' it brought tears to her eyes. 'But that was okay,' Eve recalled. 'The important thing was that she recognized my sense of loss. I was very touched by her sympathy.'

Ellen was less fortunate when she called her brother following an early loss in a pregnancy that would have been due at Christmas:

> He said that was a terrible time to have a baby anyway because kids who have birthdays near Christmas always get cheated on presents. I know he was trying to make me feel better, but I just wanted to scream at him that I would have welcomed a baby at any time of the year.

Loved ones may also fail to respect the choices you make about honouring your baby with a name or a religious ritual, even if they support you in other ways. Adele's brother was in close touch with her following each of her two losses, but when he discovered that she had named her second child, he objected. 'I thought you would have learned after the first one and not bothered to name the second one,' he told his sister. 'I did learn,' Adele replied. 'I learned you need to name your children.'

Chance encounters with people you care about can be just as disappointing and awkward, especially if they occur in a public place. Annette and her husband ran into close friends on the street shortly after her early miscarriage. Their friends already knew about the loss, but this was the first time they had met face-to-face. 'The woman said to me, "I heard what happened to you,"' recalled Annette. 'Then she visibly shuddered and said "Yuck!" The four of us were frozen there, not able to say anything.'

Tactless comments from people you do not know well can be even more enraging. In some situations you may feel so blatantly angry about a person's response that you blurt out the first thing that comes to mind, even if it seems equally thoughtless or rude. Ellen attended a company picnic where she encountered the wife of one of her husband's employees:

> I barely knew this woman, but she came up to me and said, 'I just heard about your most recent miscarriage. My God, what are you going to do, adopt?' 'That's none of your business!' I snapped at her as I went back to spooning potato salad onto my plate.

Some grieving parents are caught completely off guard by calls from vendors selling baby products. Nappy service companies, baby photographers, and the like can descend on unsuspecting parents after a loss, assuming that all went well with the pregnancy. Molly was upset by solicitations she received after her baby was stillborn, but found a way to cope with the onslaught:

> When one saleswoman opened the conversation with 'How's your new baby?' I simply said, 'My baby is dead.' I felt it was okay to shock them a little, and I didn't feel guilty about directing my anger toward them, since I didn't care about these people. I actually appreciated the opportunity to try to educate them about pregnancy loss, explaining that everything doesn't always go perfectly.

Your friends and family may also err by assuming you don't want to talk about the loss because it will be too painful for you, so they avoid mentioning it at all. In fact, this lack of response can be especially difficult to handle.

Molly found it hard to bear when people avoided her out of embarrassment or said nothing about her loss when they did eventually encounter her:

Some friends are no longer friends because they thought we didn't want to talk about our baby. The pain we felt when people ignored our loss was terrible. For us, it was another way of ignoring our son, whose existence we desperately needed to acknowledge.

Try not to be overly concerned if you have occasional angry outbursts when people say the wrong thing or ignore your sorrow by saying nothing. Once people who care about you understand your situation, they can usually absorb both your anger and their own embarrassment. Although such encounters can create a gulf of disappointment and rage between you and others, if this happens in a relationship you value, you can always call the person to explain your response when you are feeling better.

A few weeks after her friend had said 'Yuck' to her, Annette spoke with the same woman by phone and explained why she had become so silent after their encounter. 'She apologized for having been so tactless and really showed much more sympathy this time,' Annette recalled. 'After that conversation, a lot of my anger toward her dissipated.'

You may derive a sense of accomplishment by confronting people whose responses are inconsiderate, when you feel up to it. Thoughtless comments or silences present an opportunity to educate others about pregnancy loss and how it should be handled in our society. 'I felt so passionately about telling people how important it was to make a connection to us in our grief,' said one bereaved mother, 'it became almost a crusade for me.'

Coping With Social Pressures

After the initial shock of your news has worn off, people usually expect you to recover fairly quickly. You may feel frustrated by having to respond to social pressures to get on with your life, especially if you face decisions that continue to remind you of your loss.

If your pregnancy had advanced far enough so friends gave you baby gifts before your loss, you may be wondering what to do with them. The presents may remain in boxes in what would have been the baby's room, a sad reminder of the loss. It is important to keep in mind that this was still your pregnancy and your baby. Try to find the approach that makes you feel more comfortable and that honours your memories of the baby as well as your future plans for a family.

Linda was still in her twenties and her first pregnancy had progressed normally, so she welcomed baby presents from friends and coworkers. She was about halfway through her thank you cards when her son was born, only to die four hours later:

> It was difficult to continue with the remainder of the thank you notes, but I wrote to people saying that I hoped my next baby would enjoy the gift, or explained that I was keeping the present because I was not going to give up on having children. I didn't want to return any of the gifts because I knew I would have a baby by some means. What would my friends have done with the returned gifts anyway? It may have been more painful for them to get them back, too.

If your baby was born gravely ill before you experienced your loss, you may have been subjected to a different set of disconcerting responses from others. The conventional congratulations and customs surrounding a normal birth may have seemed empty and insincere.

Amelia was saddened by the flower arrangements friends sent when her baby daughter, who eventually died, was born three months prematurely. 'They sent the traditional bouquet, with a vase in the shape of a pink baby shoe, that I associated with feeling happy and congratulatory,' she explained. 'A critically ill baby is not a joyous event.'

If your baby was very ill at birth, you may have wondered if sending out birth announcements was appropriate. Many parents have found that a simple handwritten note on a plain piece of stationery is more in keeping with their mood and the actual news about their baby. You may have been equally uncertain how to respond to gifts you received, especially items of clothing meant for an older, healthy baby.

One option is simply not to respond to the gifts. Once the baby has died, most people would not expect a response, and if they don't understand, let it be their problem, not yours. As one bereaved mother who did not send thank you notes decided, 'It was a time when I had to give myself some kind of a break. I needed to forgive myself for changing the rules of etiquette a bit.'

When family and friends do come through with thoughtful gifts for gravely ill newborns, your gratitude may extend beyond your baby's death. Perhaps such caring people gave you the opportunity to suggest an appropriate gift, or they had experienced a similar situation themselves, or had good instincts. Amelia appreciated a little brass picture frame she received from a friend who had suffered her own losses:

> We put a photo of Olivia in there immediately, while she was still in

hospital. It was so appropriate, because it was a gift that acknowledged the baby she was and the important person she was to us. That little framed picture became even more meaningful after Olivia died.

You may find that family members and friends who talked about the loss in the beginning become less willing to listen after some time has passed. It may be difficult for you to bring up the subject weeks or months after the loss, even though you and your partner still feel the need to talk about it. Loved ones who cannot sustain the same responsiveness for subsequent losses that they showed for your initial loss may also disappoint you. One mother who suffered several first-trimester miscarriages remarked that after her first loss people sent flowers and little notes of condolence. But her second and third losses were greeted by total silence. 'It was as if they didn't know what to do with me, if I was going to keep losing babies and demand their sympathy,' she recalled.

In the hope of healing more quickly without the thoughtless comments of others, you and your partner may close in on yourselves. But this message can backfire if it is inadvertently communicated to friends and family who then decide not to reach out to you. They may stop calling or visiting when you still need to know that others remember and care about your loss.

You may also begin to perceive that some people don't want to be near you, as if pregnancy loss were communicable, or at least unlucky. This 'jinx mentality' may seem especially strong if you live in a community where large families are the norm and you are surrounded by pregnant women. After her second miscarriage, Virginia went to a community centre she frequented in her town. 'I felt I started losing friends there because pregnant women didn't want to bother with me,' she admitted. 'I was the failure, the one who couldn't have a second child. I seemed to frighten them.'

Both you and your loved ones probably feel unprepared to grapple with these painful encounters. Silence drops over your conversations, while embarrassment replaces the comfort you need from people you know care for you. One father found that he had to keep reminding himself that people just didn't know what to say. 'I wonder if my response toward a friend's pregnancy loss would be appropriate, without having experienced a loss myself,' he confessed. Try not to take hurtful remarks personally, but if someone's thoughtless comments make you angry, this is completely understandable.

When your friends and family don't offer the solace you crave, the result is an isolation that can fuel depression and inhibit appropriate grieving.

This is why outside help, especially that provided by a pregnancy loss support group, can enable you to grieve properly. Appendix D can help you locate a pregnancy loss support group near you.

Being With Pregnant Women and Little Children

Immediately after your loss, you may be able to sequester yourself from the outside world, staying home as much as you need. Eventually you must venture out again, first on short errands, and ultimately back to work or your regular routine, bringing you in touch with people who are pregnant or who have small children.

Casually visiting the children of friends and family who offered you emotional support during your ordeal may be more bearable than encountering the children of strangers. However, even these informal get-togethers can be distressing.

Shortly after one of her early losses, Vera and her husband were scheduled to visit close friends who had a newborn baby. They had planned to go out with their friends and the baby, but cold weather prompted the new parents to insist they all stay home. Vera suddenly felt trapped in their house:

> If we had been outside, there would have been distractions all around us, but we had to sit there and look directly at the baby the whole time. And all they talked about was the baby. I was on the verge of tears the entire time we were there.

One way to avert this kind of situation is to let friends with babies know in advance that you will only get together if they hire a baby-sitter and go out with you, away from the confines of their home. You may even have to explain that you can't get together at all for a while, until you are feeling better. You probably wish your friends and family would come up with these solutions by themselves, but as Vera admitted, 'Too often their excitement about their own happiness interferes with their ability to be sensitive to someone who is unhappy.'

The pressure to attend more formal and joyful events involving the children of loved ones, such as birthday parties and christenings, can be especially difficult after your loss. In addition to grappling with uncomfortable feelings of anger, resentment, and jealousy, you may fear bringing a pallor of gloom to each celebration. 'I hated the thought of being the sad person at a happy event,' lamented one mother who debated attending her nephew's christening shortly after she had experienced a miscarriage.

It is important to do what feels right and manageable, to respect your feelings and your period of bereavement. If you think an event will be too upsetting for you, excuse yourself and don't attend. Usually a reminder of your circumstances will help the hosts understand and respect your decision. You might say something like, 'I appreciate the invitation, but I'm still feeling sad about my loss and I'm not up to going to a party.' If you are uncomfortable explaining this, ask a close friend or relative to express your regrets.

Once you open up about your feelings, people's compassion may surprise you. Annette recalled feeling pressured by her sister-in-law to attend her niece's first birthday party, which occurred shortly after Annette's early miscarriage:

> We didn't go, and I even refused to look at the pictures of the party when we visited my sister-in-law a couple of weeks later. She was not offended at all and really seemed to understand my feelings, for which I was truly grateful.

If you decide to attend an event, allow yourself to leave early if you become too uncomfortable. One woman who had just suffered a midterm loss agonized over an invitation to her cousin's forthcoming wedding. When she couldn't decide what to do, she brought it up in a support group she was attending at the time:

> The people in my group said I had permission not to attend, or that if I went, I could leave any time I couldn't handle the pressure. Just knowing I could leave actually enabled me to stay through the entire wedding, even the reception.

Although you can't avoid every potentially distressing situation, you may be able to handle your expressions of jealousy or grief by allowing yourself a period of time after your loss when you do not arrange gatherings or attend celebrations with friends or relatives who are either pregnant or have small children. It may just be too upsetting to socialize when you feel envious of someone you care for, and angry because they have what you don't. It is exhausting to look friendly and polite when you are hurting and grieving in the face of their joy.

While you may be able to remove yourself from most situations where being with pregnant women or babies proves extremely difficult, it is harder to cope when pregnancies occur within your immediate family. Wendy gave birth to a daughter who died two weeks later while her sister was still in the early stages of her own pregnancy. Wendy found herself facing her sister's advancing pregnancy while grieving her own loss. 'I hated her for having what I didn't have,' conceded Wendy, 'and then I hated myself for hating her.'

You may also begin to feel guilty that your loss has somehow altered your loved ones' perceptions of pregnancy. Wendy felt that having given birth to a baby with a fatal congenital defect affected her sister's experience of her own pregnancy by making her unnecessarily worried:

> It was as if my sister were suddenly aware of everything that could go wrong. I felt as if I had taken away her innocence and joy about pregnancy. And I felt I had been responsible for making her feel guilty about having something I so desperately wanted. It was very hard for me on so many levels.

The intensity of your anger, guilt, and jealousy can be so extreme you may begin to doubt you will ever recover some of your relationships with family and friends. Some bereaved parents do lose friendships following a loss, or become temporarily estranged from even close family members. Amelia was afraid she would become 'this bitter, hardened woman' because her feelings of resentment toward friends and relatives with children were so strong. 'I thought my jealousy of others would seal me off from people for the rest of my life,' she said, 'I did feel better eventually, but I also formed new friendships with other couples we met who had similar losses.'

Time does help. You will eventually feel better, especially if you give your anger and jealousy outlets that allow you to talk about these natural responses to losing a pregnancy. Gulfs can be breached, wounds healed, and a new appreciation for friends and family can emerge from your loss.

What Can Help When You Turn to Family and Friends

You and your partner may have found a comforting seclusion in your home immediately after your loss, but eventually you have to face the outside world. Although you need support and may want to reach out to people, telling friends and family about the loss may be agonizing for you.

Once you start to inform people of your tragedy, you might also have to grapple with their lack of understanding. Well-intentioned but hurtful remarks may leave you angry and embittered. Friends and family with children may expect you to socialize with them or attend events that involve their youngsters, as if nothing had happened to you.

Here are some suggestions for ways to explain your tragedy that can bring you as much consolation as possible, no matter how awkward and uncomfortable your news makes people feel:

- Try to let others know that you need help, especially in the early weeks after your loss. Friends and family are often relieved if they can respond to a specific request when they otherwise wouldn't know what to do or say.
- Try not to be overly concerned about disappointing loved ones you know will be saddened by your news. It is vital that you reach out to others during this sad time.
- Consider planning how you will phrase the news of your loss to colleagues and acquaintances, so your words are as simple and straightforward as possible. Respect your need to tell people you can't discuss the loss in detail if you are too emotional at the time.
- Allow your feelings of upset to surface if someone makes an inappropriate remark. Some bereaved parents are comforted by taking this opportunity to educate others about pregnancy loss, telling them how they could respond more helpfully.
- Consider telling pregnant couples and people with small children that it is difficult to socialize with them immediately after your loss, even if they are close family or friends. If you feel you can't attend formal celebrations because you are too emotionally raw, send your regrets. Relatives and friends who truly support you and care for you will probably understand.

The Five Worst Comments You Might Hear

'It happened for the best.' No matter what the cause of your loss, it is unlikely you believe it happened for the best. This statement negates your sorrow and can make you feel you don't have a right to be sad.

What you can say in response: 'I know you mean to be comforting, but I don't think bad things ever happen to people for the best.'

'*Don't worry, you can have another baby.*' You need to mourn the baby you lost. Children are not replaceable. Also, if the mother is over thirty-five, or if you or your partner have medical or infertility problems, you may not be at all certain you *can* have another baby.

What you can say in response: 'I'm still very sad about losing this particular baby, who meant so much to me.'

'You didn't really know the baby, so it's not like losing a child who has lived with you a while.' Although there is indeed a distinction between these two losses, it is not a comforting comment. You have lost the dream of having that particular child and the expectation of being parents to that child. Although your loss may be *different* from losing an older child, it should never be deemed unworthy of grief.

What you can say in response: 'I'm sad *because* I will never know this baby I lost.'

'I know exactly how you feel.' Unless the friend or relative has been through a similar loss, this phrase may ring false and can leave you feeling angry. People cannot automatically know how other people feel, and you probably wished they had asked you how you felt instead.

What you can say in response: 'I don't think anyone can really know what I'm going through right now.'

'What are you going to do now?' In the immediate days and weeks following your loss, you are probably too stunned by your tragedy to make definite plans about becoming pregnant again or considering alternatives to pregnancy. This statement is an invasion of your privacy unless you volunteer a willingness to talk about it.

What you can say in response: 'I really don't feel like discussing that right now. I'd rather talk about the baby I just lost.'

Having people say nothing at all is probably the worst response imaginable. Saying nothing totally negates your loss and the impact it has on your lives. On the other hand, simply saying 'I don't know what to say' is both honest and direct and acknowledges the grieving parents' absolute sorrow.

What you can say in response: 'I realize you don't know what to say, but I wish you would acknowledge my pregnancy loss. I don't mind talking about it, and it hurts me when you ignore my loss.'

The Five Best Comments You Might Hear

'*I*'m so sorry. I know how much you wanted to have that baby.' This statement acknowledges both the sorrow of your loss and your desire to have the baby, while reinforcing your need to grieve.

'*It's okay to cry.*' This response validates your feelings and your need to release them without being embarrassed or guilty.

'*Would you like to talk about it?*' Instead of making assumptions about your reactions or focusing the conversation on their own experience, the friend or relative who responds this way offers the best support possible – a willing ear and a comforting shoulder.

'*Is there anything I can do for you?*' A willingness to help in practical ways can be very consoling. Offering to call other friends and family to tell the sad news, helping to dismantle the baby's room, or bringing you a home-cooked meal are important ways friends and family can truly help.

'*May I call you back in a few days to see how you are doing?*' One of the most painful realizations you will probably face as time passes is the sense that people no longer want to talk about your loss. Family members or close friends who assure you that they will continue to listen and comfort you in the weeks and months to come are truly loved ones.

CHAPTER 12

·················

HELPING YOUR CHILDREN AT HOME

Our four-year-old came into my bedroom after the stillbirth. I was lying in bed, depressed. 'Mummy,' she asked, 'do you want me to stay with you?' I told her I would like that very much. 'Okay,' she said, 'but you have to do something.' She told me to lie on my side in an 'S' position and crawled into the space by my tummy.

CHRISTINE

After your pregnancy loss, your children at home need and deserve to know what has happened, even though it is hard enough to take care of yourself, let alone worry about how to break the news to them. But if you talk with your children in a way that is sensitive to both their feelings and their ages, you can help the entire family accept the loss and begin to heal.

Children can experience many different feelings after a pregnancy loss. They may feel angry and cheated because their expected sibling will not be coming home; they can also feel guilty for having had mixed emotions about the baby their parents are so sad about losing. Often they are confused and alarmed when their daily routines disappear in the wake of a family crisis.

You may be tempted to hide your own emotions from your children, but this would only confuse them, as they would still pick up on your feelings. While it is natural for you to express your unrestrained sorrow in private or with your partner, it is all right for your children to see you cry sometimes. When you are tearful, you may want to explain that you are sad about the baby but otherwise are fine and that your sadness will get better soon.

Sharing your own thoughts and feelings about the baby can help your children open up and can reassure them that you accept their emotions, even if they are angry. If you avoid the subject, your youngsters may misinterpret your distress and assume they have done something to upset you.

A child's reaction to a loss can be quite different from an adult's. A preschooler may express grief through behaviour changes, such as bed-wetting after she had been toilet-trained, or an older child's school performance might decline. Children sometimes have nightmares or become withdrawn and depressed, experiencing your sadness as rejection and 'proof' that they are not good enough or important enough to prevent your grief. On the other hand, young children in particular may become silly and overactive, even giggling when family members talk or cry about the baby. Silly behaviour or giggling can be disconcerting if you do not realize these are uncontrollable outbursts of anxiety, not happiness.

Children do not have the same tolerance for feeling sad that grown-ups have. Youngsters may be playful and involved in their usual activities much of the time, expressing anger, anxiety, or sadness only occasionally. This is not because they are unfeeling, but because they may play and feel sad at the same time. They might also recover more quickly or simply need a break from feeling sad. As long as unexpressed feelings are not being held in or masked over, your children's return to their usual mood and activities is fine.

Sometimes children feel guilty for playing or enjoying an activity in the wake of the family's tragedy. You can reassure them that you accept and understand their behaviour by saying, 'It's okay to feel sad and still play,' or, with a hug and a smile, 'I'm glad you had a nice time at your friend's house.'

How to Talk with Your Child

Your child's reactions to your pregnancy were probably laced with both love and resentment. If the pregnancy was showing, your young child may have alternated between angrily pummelling or affectionately rubbing your growing tummy. Her anger about the potential rival for Mummy and Daddy's time can make your child fear that her negative thoughts really caused the loss. Your child may have been so excited – or indignant – about the expected birth that breaking the news can seem especially difficult. One woman's three-year-old had been very absorbed in her pregnancy, which ended in a stillbirth. 'My first thought when I learned the baby had died,' she recalled, 'was, "Whatever will I tell my son?"'

It is best to tell your child about the loss as soon as possible. If the loss occurred in the hospital, reassure her that Mother is fine, though sad about the baby, and that she will be home soon. If your loss has a known cause, share the information in simple and direct terms, since a young child's imagination can make her far more anxious than knowing the facts. Depending on the circumstances, you may want to say something like, 'The baby's lungs were not working right' or 'The baby's body did not grow properly from the very beginning, so he died.'

Florence explained how her husband broke the news of their baby's stillbirth to their three children, aged four, seven, and eight:

> He told the children the baby had died, that the cord had wrapped around her neck and she couldn't breathe. He told them I was fine. He kept it truthful but simple.

Let your youngster's questions guide you as to how much detail to give. If your child listens to your explanation and asks nothing more, you have probably said as much as she can absorb for the time being. An older child is likely to want more concrete information. She may ask when the problem happened or why the doctor couldn't save the baby. Do your best to be frank with your answers: 'We think the cord wrapped around the baby's neck a week before she was born, when I noticed she had stopped moving,' or 'When the baby was born she was no longer alive. There was nothing the doctor could do.' If the cause is unknown, be honest about this as well, explaining that sometimes even doctors don't know exactly why babies die.

Since a child of any age may blame herself for the loss, reassure your child that nothing anybody thought or did caused your loss. You might say, 'Most kids feel both happy *and* jealous when a new baby is coming. Then if the baby dies, they can worry that their jealous thoughts hurt the baby. But *nobody's* thoughts or wishes can hurt a baby. The only reason the baby died is because his body didn't work properly.'

You may find that reading children's books on loss and grief with your youngster gives the child words and permission for her feelings and helps you understand your child's experience as well. *Thumpy's Story*, by Nancy C. Dodge, is a book geared for preschool and primary children. It tells about the death of a newborn in a rabbit family and depicts with sensitivity the emotions of a sibling. The story also portrays the healing process that ultimately takes place as the family grieves and recovers yet still remembers the baby. *Thumpy's Story* is available from SANDS, whose address is listed in Appendix D.

You may be equipped to reach out to your child, and help with her feelings and fears, if you understand the special concerns and vulnerabilities of youngsters at different ages.

Toddlers and Preschoolers

Your very young child may have some awareness of both your pregnancy and loss but will not understand the permanence of death or the concept of 'forever'. He needs help in understanding what it means that the baby has died and can never come back, a concept your child may grasp only gradually. You can help by explaining the loss in terms your child can understand and by responding patiently to his repeated questions. One mother explained her miscarriage to her preschooler by reminding him of a nature project he had done. He had planted several seeds in a cup of earth; some germinated, but several did not. The mother told him her miscarriage was like one of the seeds that had not sprouted, an explanation he was able to understand and accept. You can use other examples from your child's experience, such as the death of a family pet, or a baby bird who has fallen out of its nest, to help explain the finality of a pregnancy loss.

One expert in family bereavement, suggests explaining to the child that 'dead' means that the body doesn't work anymore, that the baby cannot move, cry, see, eat, or feel anything, including heat, cold, or pain. Even in the face of these explanations, your young child may continue to ask if the baby will be coming home. Be patient and consistent with your answers, and gradually, as the child absorbs your explanations and matures, he will come to understand the permanence of the loss.

Six months after having a stillborn baby, one father found his two-year-old son looking through drawers in the 'baby's room' for the baby:

> We talked to him and told him the baby would not be coming. When he was three he started to understand. Every year we light a candle in church, or do something special to commemorate the baby. So now he knows.

Since your young child will take explanations literally, it is important to avoid euphemisms such as 'We lost the baby,' 'The baby went away,' 'Being dead is like being asleep,' or 'God took him for an angel.' To your preschooler, something that is lost can be found and someone who goes away can come back. If being dead is like being asleep, your youngster may become fearful of going to sleep, and if God took the baby for an angel, your child may be scared that God will take him next.

Your young child can fear for his own safety following a loss because the child's sense of security depends on the well-being of you and your partner, since you provide his physical and emotional care. When Mummy and

Daddy are upset, the child's world is threatened. He will probably react strongly to being away from either of you, so try to keep avoidable separations to a minimum.

Your preschooler can also be anxious after a pregnancy loss because he makes connections between events that are really unrelated. He may fear that since your baby died, someone else in the family will die soon, too, a thought that can make him especially worried about the safety of a hospitalized mother. Whether or not your child verbalizes these fears, it is wise to reassure him that the sickness or problem the baby died from was different from sicknesses other family members can get and that the rest of the family is going to be fine.

Don't be too concerned if your young child becomes short-tempered and prone to angry outbursts after your loss. One four-year-old boy had a friend over a few weeks after his baby brother was stillborn. One minute he was playing and seemed to be fine; then suddenly he threw himself on the ground and shouted, 'I want my baby!' While outbursts like this can be upsetting for you, your child is letting you know he feels distressed and needs comforting. With time, these displays of temper should lessen and then stop.

Your youngster may also surprise you by expressing love and concern for you with beautifully spontaneous and poignant gestures. Karen became depressed after a miscarriage and was touched when her two-and-a-half-year-old daughter responded to her mood. 'I was lying down and she came over to me and said, "Mummy, are you having a hard day?"' Karen recalled, 'and then she put her security blanket on me to comfort me.'

You can help your preschool child adjust to a pregnancy loss by giving him lots of attention and care. Tell your child that you love him and that you are going to be fine. With your help, he can feel reassured that while the expected baby has died, the sadness at home will get better, and he is safe, valued, and loved.

Children Aged Six to Eleven

Our seven-year-old thought she had caused the stillbirth. Before the delivery, she had a dream that the baby had died. One day she got very upset and finally asked us, 'Do you hate me because I made the baby die?' We explained to her that nothing she thought about or wished for could cause a death.

FLORENCE

Between the ages of about six and nine, a child will begin to understand the finality of death, a concept that can be abruptly brought home following a pregnancy loss. Younger children often look on death as a *taker*, something violent that comes and gets you, like a burglar or a ghost.

Florence noticed that her eight-year-old daughter seemed to understand the loss better than her younger siblings:

> Rosemary knows something that dies will never come back. She had a pet gerbil she was very attached to and it died. We got her another one, but it wasn't the same thing. Her younger sister thinks, 'If Mum gets another baby things will be fine.' Rosemary knows another baby won't replace our baby who died.
>
> The pregnancy loss was thrust upon Rosemary, and she was forced to accept death. To her, having to accept death was as difficult as losing the baby.

Allowing your child to express a full range of emotions can help her overcome anxieties. Ellen was shocked at first when she told her six-year-old son she had suffered a miscarriage, and he blurted out, 'I didn't want a baby anyway!' He complained that he dreaded visits from a neighbour's baby, who ruined his drawings and Lego creations. Ellen assured him she understood his feelings but reminded him that when his little sister had been that age, they used to put his creations out of her reach. 'I do remember that!' he said. Ellen also pointed out what an adoring sibling and great playmate his sister had become. This discussion allowed her son's mixed feelings to surface, instead of only negative ones that could have left him guilty and afraid of his 'destructive' wishes.

Younger children may show anger or anxiety by picking fights with siblings and schoolmates or by challenging their parents' and teachers' authority. You may want to let your child's teacher know about your loss and keep in close contact with her, to make sure your child's behaviour has not changed at school even if the child seems fine at home.

Your child might become very protective of you after your loss. Florence recalled how her eight-year-old sprang to her defence for months when anyone mentioned their stillborn baby:

> My oldest daughter got upset with people who talked about the loss because she thought it would upset me. If someone mentioned the baby and my eyes got teary, she would say, 'That was really clever, now look what you've done!'

You will probably feel grateful for your child's obvious love and concern when she attempts to keep you from feeling sad. At the same time, you may want to remind her that while you are sometimes unhappy about the baby, you are fine, and that little by little you will feel better.

Because your school-age child is learning so much about her world, she may be interested in the biological details of what happened, such as what part of the baby's body stopped working and why. If you have information about medical causes for your loss, share them with your child, using her questions as a guide for how much detail to give.

Like other children her age, your child is also in the process of developing a sense of right and wrong, morality, and fairness. The death of an infant can greatly upset the child's sense of justice and order in the world, and you may find yourself struggling to explain the loss.

Florence had no ready reply to her daughter's pointed questions about her stillborn sister: 'The baby was so young, Mum, she never hurt anybody. Why did she have to die?' Florence could only answer, truthfully, 'I don't really know why. There isn't a reason for everything. We all have trouble understanding why it happened.'

There may be no simple answers you can give your youngster who is struggling with the difficult notions of justice and injustice in the world, and the realization that death is an inevitable – and irreversible – part of life. You can foster trust by honestly sharing your own emotional struggles, upset, and strength, and you can show by your example how much family relationships mean at a time of loss.

Preteens and Teenagers

Your adolescent child will not need help understanding what death means – he knows it is inescapable and irrevocable. But a pregnancy loss can be very painful to your teenager, who is already struggling with the mood swings and feelings of vulnerability that go hand in hand with the adolescent years.

Since many families who have teenagers when a pregnancy loss occurs are remarried families, your adolescent may already have been burdened with complicated feelings about the pregnancy. He may have felt jealous or torn by conflicting loyalties, or might have hoped the baby would firmly unite the tentative bonds within your newly blended family.

Confronted with a pregnancy loss, your adolescent may feel his world has been turned upside down. Angry, guilty, and helpless, maybe embarrassed by having to acknowledge his parents' sexuality, an adolescent may be overwhelmed by the loss and by his own emotional tumult. Your teenager may also believe the loss is a punishment for his ambivalent feelings about the baby.

Your teenager needs help and support in understanding and accepting his anger and sorrow over your pregnancy loss. Since it is natural for teens to be concerned with their image, your adolescent may hate to cry and might consequently develop physical symptoms instead, such as headaches, stomach pains, or sleeping too little or too much.

Try to talk with your teenager honestly about your sadness and anger over the loss without being afraid to show your feelings or tears. Whether your teenager had expressed excitement or ambivalence about the pregnancy, talk over the hopes or anxieties he shared with you and how the loss has changed your plans. You might recall with your teenager, 'We talked together for so many months about having a new baby, and you worked so hard with Dad getting the room ready. It's hard to believe after all those hopes and all that work that the baby died,' or 'I know it was difficult for you to get used to the idea that a new baby was going to come into our family. But even though you were worried about it, I can see how upset you are that the baby died.'

Recalling the plans and fears you and your teenager shared during the pregnancy, as well as the shock of the loss, can open up discussions and help your adolescent accept his ambivalence and grieve the lost possibilities and the baby who has died.

Be on guard if your adolescent seems unable to talk about his upset and instead seeks relief through the use of alcohol, drugs, or sexual activity. These behaviours can be perilous and can block the grieving process. If you are concerned that your teenager is using these risky outlets to relieve stress, by all means seek professional advice.

Special Issues for You to Consider

No matter how old your other children may be, you will face practical issues together following your pregnancy loss. In the case of midterm or late losses, you may need to address your children's desire to see their baby brother or sister and say goodbye. You may wonder if it is appropriate for them to participate in religious rituals or how to help them tell their friends and peers about the loss.

Saying Goodbye to a Baby Sibling

You may be uncertain at what age it is beneficial, rather than frightening, for your child to see and say goodbye to a dying or deceased baby sibling. This decision is a very individual one and depends on the needs and maturity of your child. Families with children as young as four have found that their youngsters expressed a strong wish to see a dying or deceased infant sibling. If your child wants to see the baby and you think she can handle it, it is important to explain the death and describe the baby's appearance before gently giving your child the choice.

Oliver remembered when his five-year-old daughter, Kate, insisted on seeing her brother who had died one hour after his premature delivery:

> After the baby died I went to Kate's school and brought her to the hospital. My wife was holding the baby. Kate looked at him, touched him, held him, got to know him in a way. She cried. Over the next six months she would break out crying occasionally; otherwise she was fine. I feel it really helped her to say goodbye to the baby.

If your child did not see her baby sibling, you can help the child to accept and mourn the loss by showing her a picture of the baby or the baby's footprints, or, if you saw the baby, by telling your child what the infant looked like. Your young child may want to draw pictures or make clay models of a baby, whether or not she saw the infant. By showing interest in your child's creations and letting her talk about them, you convey acceptance of your child's feelings. Your child's expression of emotions through art, talking, and play are all healthy efforts to accept the reality of a confusing and upsetting loss.

Mementoes can help a child born after the pregnancy loss understand who her baby sibling was. Amelia explained how she envisioned telling her son about his sister, who died in infancy two years before he was born. 'My husband and I have already discussed it and agreed that we will tell Jacob about his sister,' she revealed. 'Someday I'd like to show Jacob his sister's album filled with pictures from her brief life.'

Your Child and Religious Rituals

If you find solace in religion, this is a time when you may want to share your faith with your child. It does not help to mouth a doctrine you do not believe yourself, as children of any age will sense this. However, by expressing true religious convictions, you can share with your child the comfort these beliefs give to you.

If you want to convey your belief in the afterlife of the baby's spirit, it is important to acknowledge the finality of physical death. Otherwise a young child might think the baby is physically alive somewhere and able to return.

If you decide to hold a ritual for your baby, you may feel unsure if it will be helpful or upsetting for other siblings to attend. One expert suggests that children of four or five and older be given the choice to attend a funeral, memorial service, or burial for the baby, because 'The funeral is a rite of separation . . . the bad dream is real.   . . It is an opportunity to say goodbye.' Children of primary age and older are likely to be concerned about having proper ceremonies for the baby and may insist upon attending.

If your child wishes to attend and you feel comfortable about having him there, it is helpful to tell your child in detail what to expect. Tell him about the appearance of the room, who will be there, the likelihood that some people will cry, what the service will consist of, and how long it will be. Consider arranging for your child to sit with someone he knows well who can go out with the child if he wants to leave early. You can ask your child if he would like to give a gift to be placed in the coffin, such as a flower, or toy of his choice.

It is important for your child to be allowed to change his mind about attending a funeral service, even at the last minute. You might want to invite a friend or relative your child trusts to be available that day, just in case the child suddenly decides to stay home.

If you have an adolescent, he will probably benefit from attending any religious rituals you observe. By including your teenager, you convey that sadness is an acceptable emotion and that a funeral is an appropriate time and place for the release of grief. Rituals can give your teenager an opportunity to say goodbye to the baby and to accept the finality of the loss while providing the comforting presence of family and friends.

Your Child's Peers

Your child's friends may not know how to act toward her when your family is deprived of an expected sibling. But with your guidance and encouragement, and with the help of social customs and rituals, young friends can learn to express sympathy for your bereaved child in ways that are meaningful and sustaining.

One sensitive primary school teacher suggested that each classmate write a note of condolence to Luke, whose baby brother had died shortly after an emergency delivery. Months after the loss, Luke still talked about those notes, especially one of his favourites, a heartfelt but humorous limerick written by a classmate:

> Once Luke's mother gave birth to a brother.
> It didn't come out so she gave a shout,
> But maybe she'll have another.
> Your pal, BRIAN

Christine, whose baby was stillborn, found the religious rituals her family observed provided an opportunity for the friends of her four surviving children to demonstrate sympathy for her bereaved youngsters:

> We had a burial, coffin, grave. We had an obituary, and a special Mass was offered. It was wonderful for the children. Their friends came and they all cried together. They felt the peer support keenly.

Once you have helped establish communication between your child and her friends about your loss, you may also notice that the youngster has an increased empathy for the grief of others. One little boy, whose premature baby brother had died, invited over a friend who had recently lost his father. The little host's mother was amazed and touched at how the boys related their losses:

> They sat together, talking at dinner like little adults. The friend talked about his deceased father. My son said, 'I know what it's like. My brother died.'

After the Crisis

Children of any age derive a sense of security from their regular, predictable routines. A pregnancy loss, with separation from one or both parents, visits from family and friends, and everybody's emotional upset, throws a family's – and a child's – usual schedule into upheaval.

While your child may continue to have questions or worries about your pregnancy loss for weeks or months after, you can help her regain a sense of security by restoring her routine as soon as possible after the loss. Perhaps you can pack your child's lunch or help with homework, if this is what she is used to. Keeping to the same bedtime rituals, such as reading a story and having the regular lights-out time, also helps.

You may find that caring for your surviving child helps you as much as it helps her, that the child's love and need for you reaffirm your role as a parent. When you feel ready, you may even want to plan some special activities with your child that can help both of you to heal emotionally.

Ellen had her fourth miscarriage only three days before her son started nursery. After the loss, she volunteered to do an art project with his class that was so successful she continued the activity through the school term. 'My son loved having me in his classroom,' Ellen remembered, 'and I enjoyed getting to know his teacher and classmates. It was such a positive channel for me after the loss, and it helped him, too.'

It is important for you to have adequate support for yourself as you mourn, so you can help your surviving child. For mothers especially, it is difficult to deal with a child's anxiety or anger when you are upset and physically depleted. Accept any extra available help – from partner, relatives, or babysitters – to ease the stresses during the early weeks after your loss. This extra support can enable you to give full attention, for periods of time, to your child's emotional needs. 'You have to take care of yourself,' one bereaved mother expressed. 'Otherwise I believe it will backfire later.'

A youngster needs time to understand what a pregnancy loss means and to absorb her own feelings about it. You can help by keeping the lines of communication open. A young child in particular will often ask the same questions over and over, or as time passes, will come up with new questions. This process, which can go on for months, reflects the child's efforts to assimilate the reality of your family's loss.

You will have many opportunities to help your child adjust to a loss. Just as your youngster may need to repeat a question, you also may want to go back and reopen a discussion about what happened, or about your child's feelings and worries. Choose a relaxed time other than bedtime, perhaps while sitting with your child for an afternoon snack or while taking a drive together. You can recall aloud, 'Remember how we used to talk about the baby when we were driving places, thinking what it would be like to have him along? I still think about him at times like this. Do you sometimes think about him, too?' Sharing your own thoughts and feelings about the baby can help your child open up as well, allowing you to convey acceptance of her feelings, whatever they may be.

If You and Your Family Need Extra Help

Your child's reactions will depend on his age and personality, on the circumstances of the loss, and on your own grief responses. It is common for a child to experience both physical symptoms and behaviour changes after a pregnancy loss in the family.

In most cases, a child's symptoms will diminish and behaviour changes will disappear over a few weeks or months. But sometimes behaviour changes, either at home or at school, continue without showing signs of improvement. This can happen for many different reasons, and when it does occur, it is wise to seek professional help.

It is natural for you to be consumed by your own grief after a pregnancy loss. And it may be especially difficult, in the early weeks after a loss, to respond to the demands of your child. For some parents this difficulty persists, and the child begins to react to the changes in routine and to the parents' lack of involvement with him.

Ginny and her husband had a healthy son, Warren, followed by two early losses and a stillbirth. After the third loss, her husband withdrew emotionally for several months.

Having lost three pregnancies, and with inadequate support from her family, Ginny became very depressed. Sometimes she resented Warren for surviving when the other babies didn't. Her relationship with her son suffered. 'I was ignoring Warren,' she recalled. 'I wasn't taking him to the park or anything. I stayed in bed all day, so he just had to watch TV.'

Understandably, with his mother depressed and his father emotionally unavailable. Warren's behaviour changed, and in ways Ginny found hard to take in a five-year-old. 'He cried with no explanation and wouldn't say what was wrong,' Ginny explained. 'He made a fuss about everything, like taking a bath or going to bed.'

After these difficulties went on for several months, Ginny finally went to her priest for help, which was a turning point for both her and Warren:

> My priest helped me to realize that I was paying more time and attention to the babies who died than to the child I had. This helped me start to accept the losses more. I started to feel so grateful for my son.
>
> Afterward I noticed a change in Warren. He got better after I changed toward him.

A pregnancy loss can have a traumatic aftermath for a child if he witnessed emergency medical procedures or if his mother's life was endangered. Eight-year-old Luke saw his mother go into full-term labour late at night. Five minutes later, she went into shock and collapsed due to separation of the placenta from the uterine wall. While the ambulance rushed his mother and father to the hospital, Luke followed in a police car, sirens blaring.

After the emergency delivery, Luke overheard doctors saying his mother had a fifty-fifty chance of survival and that the baby's chances were even less. His mother recovered, but the baby died.

Not surprisingly, Luke's mother noticed behaviour changes that lingered long after these frightening events:

> A few months after the loss, Luke was almost eruptive. His temper peaked quickly; he had a short fuse. He got frustrated more easily than before. If his drawing wasn't going well, he threw down his pen. He was more aggressive than we had ever seen before.

Six months after the loss, Luke's parents consulted a family therapist on how they could help their son with his distress. The professional encouraged them to talk openly with Luke about the loss and his mother's medical crisis, so he could share his own feelings and fears. Luke's behaviour gradually improved.

If your loss involved a medical emergency, you can help your child by talking about what happened, by giving realistic assurances about the danger having passed, and by giving the child opportunities to express what these events were like for him. Children are emotionally resilient, and with your help, and professional support if needed, your youngster should gradually come to terms with your pregnancy loss and return to his usual behaviours, activities, and interests.

What Can Help Your Children After a Loss

Dealing with your child's response to your pregnancy loss can be very taxing when you are in the midst of your own grief. It is natural for children of all ages to experience mood and behaviour changes after a pregnancy loss in the family. You can help your child by explaining the loss in simple, frank terms and by being truthful about your own sorrow. If you are sensitive to the child's feelings and anxieties, she should gradually come to terms with the loss.

Here are some suggestions that can enable you to help your child after a pregnancy loss:

- Tell your child about the loss as soon as possible, simply and directly. Try to avoid euphemisms such as 'The baby is sleeping' or 'We lost the baby,' since a young child in particular may take these statements literally and may fear going to sleep or expect the baby to be found.
- Your youngster might feel sad and vulnerable after your loss and needs lots of love and attention. Parents, other relatives, close friends, and babysitters can all help.
- Assure your child that nothing she or anyone else thought about, said, or did caused the pregnancy loss. Explain that the rest of the family is fine and that the sickness the baby died from is different from other sicknesses.
- If you hold a funeral service or other ritual for the baby, and if your child wishes to attend, you may want to give her that option. Children four and older are more likely to show an interest in these rituals, but again, this is very individual.
- Try to get your child's routine back to normal as soon as possible. Planning special time or activities together, when you feel ready, can help both of you during this difficult period.
- Be prepared for your child to ask the same questions over and over, or for different questions to arise as she grows and matures. Try to respond to your child's concerns so the child feels free to talk about this significant event in her life.
- If your child has symptoms or behaviour changes that continue for many weeks after a loss, the child may need additional help. Be sure you have adequate support for yourself, and consult a qualified psychotherapist if your child's difficulties continue. See Appendix D for help in locating a psychotherapist.

CHAPTER 13

FOR BEREAVED GRANDPARENTS

The initial shock was to know there was no grandchild. We had looked forward to another grandchild so much; they are so rewarding. We felt terrible.

SID

The hardest thing about going through a loss with your children is the grief you feel for them, because you can't do anything. I am conditioned as a mother to fix things, make things better, and I couldn't.

MAUREEN

Grandchildren bring a treasured feeling of family continuity and a unique gratification to you, their grandparent. They often create a new and cherished bond between you and your adult children as well, so when an unborn or newborn baby dies, you grieve doubly, for yourself and for your children. It is especially difficult for you to feel so helpless and sad when you see your grown children suffer.

When a pregnancy loss occurs, you may initially feel shock and disbelief that an expected family joy has turned into a tragedy. Sid was upset when his adult daughter and son each had babies die near term:

The pregnancies had really traumatic endings. It was a terrible shock; there was no way of being prepared. Then my wife and I realized this had really happened, that there was no way to go back and make it different. We had to concentrate on how we would get through it.

As a grandparent, you may not know how to respond to this family tragedy. You may have been raised with the attitude that one doesn't talk about a pregnancy loss, that one puts the loss in the past and gets on with life. If your children are openly upset after their loss, this can leave you worried and confused. You may be tempted to help by urging the young couple to have another baby, or, if they are already parents, by encouraging them to be grateful for the children they have. While well-intentioned, such comments are likely to be hurtful rather than comforting. The more you are able to accept that mourning is a painful but useful means of healing a loss, the better you can be a true aide to your bereaved children.

Your reaction to this family tragedy will be very individual and will depend on the relationship you already had with your adult children before the loss occurred. You may feel the loss deeply but wonder if you should share your grief, or if it will only further burden your bereaved children. As one grandmother expressed:

> I could cry for them, but should I, so they know how bad I feel? Or should I try to keep cool so they don't feel they've utterly disappointed me by not giving me grandchildren?

Your children will probably appreciate knowing you also feel the loss, as long as you do not expect them to be your primary source of support.

As a grandparent, you can help your bereaved children more than anyone else, a help that may permanently deepen family ties. If you have survived a pregnancy loss yourself, you may be able to reach out and sustain your children in especially meaningful ways.

Jane had experienced a miscarriage and a stillbirth as a young woman. She found that memories of her own losses resurfaced when her daughter, who suffered from infertility, became pregnant and then miscarried. Jane's ability to say she was sad, and to listen to her daughter, comforted both of them and created a closeness that helped mother and daughter cope with their grief:

> I had a lot of emotional reactions after my own miscarriage, and they all came back to me. And after my stillbirth I got all the questions, such as 'What did you have?' dying myself a little by having to answer that the baby had died.
>
> I told my daughter about my own losses. I wanted to prepare her so she would know it's a hard time emotionally. I do tell her I am sad about her baby, and for her. I talk to her at least once a week. If she's feeling low, she'll say so. I can tell if she's been crying.

Your children may ask you to dismantle the baby's room and store the baby supplies before the sad homecoming from the hospital. One grandmother had the unhappy task of going to her daughter and daughter-in-law, in turn, after each lost a newborn. When both bereaved mothers asked her to put away their baby things, the grieving grandmother recalled, 'The afternoon I packed up the second set of baby items, I thought that no grandmother should have to do this twice.'

You might want to talk over your feelings about the pregnancy loss with your spouse, relatives, or friends. If you are religious, you may wish to speak with a member of the clergy or friends from your congregation. It is especially important for you to be sustained during your bereavement so you can be strong enough to support your children.

Grandparents' Guilt

*I*f you are like many bereaved grandparents, you may suffer from feelings of guilt when your unborn or newborn grandchild dies. You may feel deeply troubled that you have lived to experience this loss. Sometimes this takes the form of 'survivor guilt,' in which you feel the order of your life has been profoundly upset, that it is somehow 'wrong' for you to be alive when a new life in the family has ended.

Painful though it may be to let your spouse or children know you feel this way, the honest sharing of feelings with your loved ones is best. Otherwise, guilt or resentment can create barriers in your family relationships when you most need to turn to one another, to share your worries and your hopes.

Pregnancy loss can be especially difficult for you if a genetic cause is suspected, as you may wonder whether you passed on the 'bad' gene.

If a genetic problem contributed to a loss, try not to be hard on yourself, as you had no control over the problem or were following your doctor's advice in an effort to protect your own pregnancy. In either case, it is important for your children to have the facts of your medical history, as advances in the early diagnosis and treatment of some genetic disorders have enhanced the chances of an eventual, successful pregnancy.

Rather than dwell on self-blame, do your best to acknowledge the problem, but then focus on emotional or practical assistance you might offer to the couple during their bereavement or if they embark on a subsequent high-risk pregnancy.

Grandmothers who had problem-free pregnancies may have a different fear, that their children will resent them for having had babies so easily. One grandmother of eight grown children wanted to be comforting to her daughter, who had miscarried three times, but questioned whether her vastly different experience would get in the way. 'Sometimes I wonder if she could be angry with me for "popping out babies" so easily,' she explained. 'I can't say "I know exactly how you feel," because I don't.'

However different your experiences with pregnancy may have been, your genuine expression of sympathy for your children's plight will probably be much appreciated. Sometimes simply saying 'Do you feel like talking?' or 'Is there anything I can do?' will allow your children to open up about their loss so that you can begin to understand their feelings and frustrations.

Even if your relationship with the bereaved couple is a close one, they may be reluctant to talk with you about their pregnancy loss to spare you their hopes and grief. One grandmother was worried that her daughter was trying to protect her, when above all the grandmother wanted to be a source of help:

> I was concerned because when my daughter had her miscarriage she didn't tell me right away. She tried to spare me. I found out from my son, who told me she had not called me right away because she had wanted me to get through the weekend undisturbed.

If your bereaved children are trying to protect you, consider letting them know that you are available to talk with them, and while you are sad, you are more concerned about them than about your own grief.

Helping Your Bereaved Children

If you visited your children during or shortly after their pregnancy loss, this was undoubtedly a very emotional time for you, but simply your presence probably meant a great deal to them. Perhaps you helped with household tasks such as shopping and cooking, or you accompanied the grieving parents to the funeral parlour, phoned relatives, or cared for other children. This assistance may have seemed insignificant to you in the face of your children's loss, but it is important and meaningful to bereaved parents who are physically and emotionally drained because of their tragedy.

If your children suffered a stillbirth or newborn death, you may have seen and held the baby with them. Your contact with the infant may have intensified your feelings of loss but might also have given you a treasured moment with your children and grandchild. Maureen spoke of how seeing her tiny granddaughter affected her grieving daughter-in-law, Tina, and herself:

I felt such grief for this baby. I saw her; she lived for four days. I told Tina how badly I felt, for her and for us.

I could tell Tina cared I was there. It meant so much to me to know I could give help and she could accept it.

If you were unable to visit your children after a pregnancy loss because of geographical distance or other constraints, it is still possible to show you care in other ways. You can acknowledge the loss with a card, flowers, or a plant, or by making a donation to a charity in memory of the baby. If there is a funeral, you may want to help with expenses if you are financially able to do so.

You can also make a point of keeping in touch through letters or telephone calls. If your children named their baby, they will appreciate your referring to your grandchild by name. Let your children know you are willing to talk about the baby when they want to, and that you are willing to talk about other things, too, when that is more comfortable for them.

Differences in opinion between you and your bereaved children can easily arise around practical decisions, such as putting away baby things, making funeral arrangements, and planning for another pregnancy. While it is natural for you to have your own wishes and views, the bereaved couple must live with their decisions and need to make these choices themselves.

Both parents and grandparents, for example, can have strong feelings about how to handle a nursery when a baby dies. When Amelia and Charles found out that their ill newborn daughter would probably be coming home soon, they quickly prepared a room for her. Afterward, when their baby died, they chose not to dismantle her room right away. To the young couple, putting away the baby things meant giving up hope of ever having a child. But Amelia's parents disagreed and, as Amelia recalled, they did not hesitate to offer their opinion:

They implied that our daughter's room should be changed into something else, like a study or guest room, and that we were weird or unhealthy to keep it as a baby's room. We resented their opinion and we resented their feeling entitled to ask us about it. It felt like an invasion of our privacy. The next time my parents came to visit, I remember locking the door to the baby's room for the first time.

In contrast, Linda turned to her mother immediately after her newborn son's death, and asked her to help store gifts that filled the baby's room:

My mother cleaned out the room and put everything in her attic so when I came home from the hospital there was nothing there. It was just an empty room with pastel curtains. I assured her I would be a parent one way or the other and that I wanted her to keep the things. She kept everything until after our next son was born. I was really grateful.

Sometimes a bereaved couple has a strong need to carry out practical arrangements themselves, while at other times they are grateful for help. In either case, it is important that the decision be theirs. If you want to help, ask your children if they would like a hand with particular tasks and let them tell you what they need.

Family Celebrations and Holidays

You will probably be part of family and holiday gatherings where the presence of babies is obviously painful for your bereaved children. As one grandmother, Maureen, recalled:

My daughter Janice and her husband came here for Christmas a few months after the death of their newborn son. Two sisters-in-law had babies the same year. It was very hard for Janice to watch these mothers with their little children.

Such family gatherings heighten the sense that a baby who should have been there is missing. This situation is terribly distressing for the bereaved couple, a fact you cannot change. However, you can quietly let the couple know that you, too, miss the baby. You can also tell your children you will understand if they want to be excused from any part of the festivities.

You can help your bereaved children by being aware that a christening, or first birthday party in the family will be difficult for them to handle in the early months after a loss. Let them know you will understand if they choose not to attend. You can offer to talk to the party's hosts, if the couple wishes, to explain their reason for declining to participate, making it clear that you respect the couple's decision. This kind of help can spare your children worry over offending relatives if your bereaved children don't want to attend.

Pregnancy After a Loss

You might have strong feelings, either positive or negative, about a future pregnancy. One grandmother confessed she hoped her son and daughter-in-law would keep trying to have children in spite of miscarriages and infertility problems. A grandfather expressed the opposite concern after both his son and daughter had losses followed by one successful birth each. 'They have good marriages and we don't want them to rock the boat,' he admitted. 'When we heard they were planning to have more children, we worried. What if something happened again?'

When another pregnancy does follow a loss, you may experience anxiety while feeling there is little you can do to help. Maureen and her husband felt apprehensive throughout the high-risk but successful subsequent pregnancies of both their daughter and daughter-in-law. 'I think they were the longest months of our lives,' Maureen admitted. 'But the end results were wonderful!'

Your anxiety over the possibility of another loss can make you wary of becoming emotionally involved with the pregnancy until the baby arrives safely. Nevertheless, you can help your children by maintaining a positive but realistic attitude about the pregnancy and by encouraging the couple with cards, letters, and telephone calls. It is all right to acknowledge your own anxiety and admit that this difficult pregnancy is tough for you, too.

Strengthening Family Ties

Pregnancy loss is a tragedy that changes a family permanently. While the loss is in no way diminished, part of the change, in the long run, can be positive. If you and your bereaved children are able to share your mutual grief, you may find your contact deeply sustaining in the distressing months after a loss. As one grandfather explained, 'We all joined forces, we were all in it together. This is what helped me and the others the most.' As you share your sorrow and rally to help one another, you may also develop richer ties and a deeper mutual appreciation.

Jane, a mother of several grown children, was geographically distant from her two daughters who had experienced miscarriages and infertility problems. But she kept in close contact and let them know of her love and concern for them. As a result, she noticed a change in her relationship to each of them:

> I feel I have more closeness with these two daughters, even though both live so far away. But somehow or other we are the really close ones, maybe for having shared all their troubles and losses.

Maureen described a positive change in her relationship to her daughter-in-law, Tina, after the death of an infant granddaughter:

> I suppose in a way I feel closer to Tina. I always felt close to her. I felt so blessed to have her for a daughter-in-law. There is even a greater bond there now, since we shared the loss.

What Can Help Bereaved Grandparents

Since your children's pregnancy loss, you may have been grieving doubly, for their pain and for the loss of your grandchild. You might feel guilty and helpless, as you are unable to protect the grieving couple from their distress.

Your love, concern, and shared sorrow, however, can be special sources of comfort to your children as they slowly put their lives back together after their loss. Here are some suggestions for getting the support you need while helping your grieving children:

- A pregnancy loss in your family may be deeply upsetting to you, as you lost a grandchild and are suffering for your own children as well. Allow yourself to talk about your feelings with your spouse, family, or friends, or within your religious community.
- Be honest about your sorrow with your bereaved children, but because of their own distress, do not expect them to be a primary source of comfort to you. Let them know you are available when they want to talk.
- If you are in a position to assist in other ways, ask how you can help, and make specific suggestions. You might offer to accompany the parents to the funeral parlour, telephone other relatives, prepare meals, shop, care for other children in the family, or help financially.
- If you live far apart and cannot visit, let the bereaved couple know you are thinking about them and the baby with telephone calls, a card, gift, or a charitable donation. If the baby was given a name,

mention it when talking about your grandchild.

- Respect the couple's decisions about putting away baby things, making funeral arrangements, and planning a subsequent pregnancy. You may have strong opinions about these matters, but the bereaved parents need to make these decisions themselves, as they must live with them.
- If a subsequent pregnancy follows the loss, let the expectant parents know you are thinking about them. Be encouraging but realistic. It is all right to let the expectant couple know this is an anxious pregnancy for you as well.
- Living through your children's pregnancy loss, and sharing the grief, can strengthen family ties and deepen your appreciation for your loved ones.

SECTION IV

SPECIAL CIRCUMSTANCES

As you begin to recover emotionally from your pregnancy loss, you and your partner may feel hopeful for the future when you return to your regular routine and start to plan for another baby. This initial sense of recovery can leave you unprepared for the impact your loss might have on other aspects of your life, such as your career or your feelings about a subsequent pregnancy. Women can find themselves unable to concentrate at work, and both men and women may discover they are unexpectedly fearful of conceiving another child. Should additional reproductive problems arise, both you and your partner may be devastated just when you thought you could begin to enjoy life again.

The following chapters will help prepare you for these issues before they arise and can enable you to find solace and validation as you struggle with the far-reaching impact your pregnancy loss can have on your life.

CHAPTER 14

THE IMPACT OF PREGNANCY LOSS ON YOUR CAREER

If you are like many bereaved mothers, your pregnancy loss affected you both personally and professionally. You may have planned a maternity leave well in advance of your due date, but cancelled the leave or turned it into a shorter one after you suffered your loss. Pregnancy and plans for motherhood may have even altered your perspective about the role of work in your life following your loss. If your future pregnancies will be high-risk, you face major decisions about how to maintain your career while putting it on hold, perhaps for a long time.

Like many women today, you may have postponed pregnancy until you were established in your career. The contrast between your professional success and the out-of-control experience of pregnancy loss can be especially frustrating. As psychiatrist Elisabeth Herz has noted, career women who lose a pregnancy are 'conditioned to set a goal, work hard toward it, and succeed.' Being faced with an ambition that may be beyond your immediate reach creates feelings of confusion and helplessness that do not fit your self-image. You may experience the normal crying spells and decreased level of work performance during bereavement as a total loss of control over your life.

Your partner, too, may react to the change in your self-image. Accustomed to seeing you as independent and accomplished, he may resent your temporary helplessness and vulnerability after your loss. One woman stopped working for several months during a difficult pregnancy that ended in a loss, and was aware how the change in her work status bothered her husband. 'He felt that a lid had been put on my development and career,' she recalled. 'He saw another loss, my loss of self-esteem, and it troubled him greatly.'

Your Career Decisions and Gratification

The leave you take from work after your loss can depend on whether you had an early miscarriage or a later loss. If you were well into the pregnancy and had already arranged a maternity leave, returning to work means an abrupt change in these plans, a shift that can be a painful reminder of your childlessness. As one mother lamented:

> I didn't know what to do about anything, my work, my leave. Should I find a new job or go back to the old one? I loved my work, but when I was pregnant with our daughter I set my mind to being at home and leaving work for a while. Then suddenly I had to go back to not being a Mum and think about work again. That was hard for me.

Your return to work after a pregnancy loss can be a very hard emotional step but one that may provide a new focus for your thoughts and energies and bring you relief after the loss. Marianne, who had three pregnancy losses, found this to be the case. 'It was very hard coming back to work, especially the second time,' she recalled. 'But going back to work was best and helped me to overcome the losses.'

If you had to put your career on hold because of your pregnancy loss, you may reach a point when you decide that having a baby will have to wait so your career can come first for a while. You might look forward to having an arena in your life where your self-esteem can blossom while you give yourself a break from the stress and possible disappointments over childbearing problems. 'After my third miscarriage I went back to college and did my M.B.A.,' explained one woman. 'I had wanted to do this for a long time, and I really needed to do something for myself.'

But this tactic can backfire. Completion of a degree or a career training programme can feel like the seal on your failure to have a baby, as if your career were a substitute for becoming a mother. Natalie enrolled in nursing college after two miscarriages and had a third loss before she completed her course. 'I thought nursing college would at least give me professional gratification, but the graduation brought home the loss,' she revealed. 'I shouldn't have graduated in May. I should have had my baby in March.'

It can be tempting to immerse yourself in work to elude the pain and grief of your loss, a tactic that may postpone but cannot prevent the mourning process. 'I used my work as an escape after the losses,' admitted Vera, who had suffered several first-trimester losses. 'I buried myself in work and repressed all my emotions, but it was unhealthy to do that.'

If you use work as an escape, you will probably discover, as Vera did, that you still need to set aside time to grieve – with your partner, in a support group, or with a psychotherapist – before you begin to feel better. Then work can become a true source of gratification rather than an evasion of grief.

A temporary decrease in career satisfaction is common after a loss. Your lack of interest in work is a normal reaction during the mourning period, when feelings of depression and disinterest can dominate your mood. Even a career that you once found prestigious and exciting can suddenly feel like just a job. A persistent longing for a child can add to your sense that work is less important than it seemed before. 'I can't shake the feeling that I should be home with a baby now and that I don't really want to be at work,' confessed Louise. 'My job is rewarding, but I want to be doing it in conjunction with the other piece of my life – the baby I want. I'm angry about work.'

Some mothers find feelings of sadness and longing for a child only recede with the birth or adoption of another baby, or through the gradual process of mourning wished-for parenthood and acceptance of an alternative life-style. Once your desire for a baby has been resolved one way or the other, your career can again feel stimulating and important.

Making decisions about your career in light of a pregnancy loss may compel you to think carefully about what is most important to you. You might discover, in the process, that your priorities have changed. You may clarify and pursue career goals that you had put on hold, or choose to cut down on professional commitments to give more time to family and friends. 'Clearly my child and family were the most important things to me,' explained Naomi, a high-powered professional who had cut back to part-time work after three miscarriages and the birth of a healthy baby. 'I might not have felt this if I hadn't had the losses.' Balancing the impact of your pregnancy loss against your career and plans for another pregnancy can leave you with a clarity of purpose whatever choices you ultimately make.

Men and Their Careers

Men usually find the importance of their careers remains unchanged or increases after a loss. Most often return to work after no leave, or a very brief one. Work can give men a welcome refuge from grief and allow them to feel helpful and productive by providing financial security for their families.

Sometimes, however, a pregnancy loss has a direct impact on a man's work or career plans. He may experience extra work pressure after a loss because of additional financial burdens due to the temporary loss of his wife's income. If he had a career change in the offing, he may feel he has to postpone or abandon his plans because of the uncertainties at home.

Jeff, a GP, whose wife had suffered three miscarriages, had been planning to start a new practice, but became concerned about the timing of this career move:

> Starting my own practice has been a goal of mine for some time. Now I have a lot of anxiety and find it scary to contemplate. My difficulty with this decision is related to the losses, in the sense that I wish our plans to have a family were secure so I could start my practice with other aspects of my life under control.

Occasionally pregnancy loss can be the impetus for a man to make a positive career change. The couple's shared loss and grief can alter his priorities so that new career decisions become possible. Eric discovered inner resources after he and his wife, Annette, lived through infertility problems followed by a pregnancy loss. When Annette then became pregnant with twins, Eric felt motivated and capable of making a significant career change to put his family on a sounder financial footing:

> I went from being a freelance writer to a computer programmer. I was a champion of Annette when she went through the infertility treatments and then the miscarriage. She was a champion for me when I went through this radical career switch. We gave each other strength because, having lived through the losses, we had learned how to do it.

Your Career Choices and High-Risk Pregnancy

I am in a never-never land now. One part of me needs a job that is challenging and absorbing so I don't feel sad all the time because I don't have a child. My whole life is set up now for having a child, and I don't have one. We are saving money for my being pregnant again and being out of work and on bed rest. I have been putting my life on hold for two and a half years.

AMELIA

When you face a future high-risk pregnancy that may include months of bed rest, you are confronted with major challenges. You are compelled to make career plans and choices based on your high-risk status, with no guarantee of motherhood. Your employment may not accommodate a leave for bed rest, or you may find it difficult to arrange coverage for your work responsibilities during your absence. Even if you are able to find and train someone to fill your job, you will probably find little appreciation from your colleagues for the complexity and difficulty of the task.

Amelia spent a great deal of time planning her leave, since she knew she would be coming back to her job and wanted it to be well-organized when she returned. 'Making all these arrangements was like having an extra job,' she remembered, 'but I felt it was my responsibility, and my colleagues expected it, too.'

You may face painful dilemmas about career opportunities that are incompatible with the care you need while pregnant. It can feel unfair to have to decide whether to make a good career move that could imperil a future pregnancy or whether to forgo career satisfaction while your reproductive future remains uncertain. Natalie was well established in a highly stressful profession when she suffered her losses, which forced her to consider the effect a future high-risk pregnancy would have on her career:

> I now have to decide whether to stay in bed for the next pregnancy; this is having a major impact on my career. I was just offered an excellent job, which I turned down because I thought it would be too stressful. With each pregnancy it is a big issue. I am so afraid that stress on the job is going to make me miscarry.

If you have worked for your employer for two years or more, and require long-term hospitalization during your pregnancy, you are entitled to take this time as sick leave, followed after the birth of your baby by the normal maternity leave. If your employer does not offer you the same job back upon your return, they can be prosecuted under the terms of the Sexual Discrimination Act. Occasionally problems can arise, if, during long-term sick leave, a pregnant woman receives statutory sick pay and as a result no longer makes sufficient National Insurance contributions required in order to be fully eligible for maternity benefits. Women who have very premature babies may be at a considerable disadvantage because maternity leave is calculated from date of delivery, and may expire before her baby leaves the hospital. The Maternity Alliance should be able to advise both employed and self-employed women about the complicated system of maternity benefits.

Even if leave for bed rest is not required, a high-risk pregnancy can still have a major impact on your work. While previously accustomed to keeping your personal life separate from work, you must inform your employer and colleagues of your pregnancy earlier than you might like. This invasion of your privacy is unfortunately necessary to ensure coverage of your work responsibilities should you suddenly have to take a leave.

It is also stressful when care for your pregnancy takes precedence over your work routine, as you take time off for medical appointments, scans and other tests. 'It was awful to have to choose between my pregnancy and my work,' recalled a financial consultant who had two previous miscarriages. 'Sometimes I would have to decide whether to get up in the middle of a client meeting, which had run late, to keep an appointment with my obstetrician.' You may find that these obligatory shifts at work have a negative effect on your status, productivity, and professional self-image.

If your career is in a male-dominated field, you can feel especially torn when a high-risk pregnancy obliges you to put the care of your unborn baby first. You probably entered your field knowing you would be under pressure to demonstrate your equal ability and productivity to your male colleagues. When your job performance is affected by a high-risk pregnancy, you can feel you are confirming the bias that men are more reliable than women in these positions, an attitude you had hoped to combat.

Tina, a research psychologist, lost a full-term pregnancy due to undiagnosed diabetes. During her next pregnancy, she was maintained on a strict regimen to stabilize her blood sugar. This required pricking her finger for a blood sugar test at regular intervals, eating meals and snacks on a frequent and strict schedule, and giving herself insulin shots at specific times throughout the day, all of which affected her career:

> I wasn't producing the way I had been; I knew it, and my boss knew it. That felt stressful, and stress makes diabetes worse. My lower pro-ductivity affected my job status, too. I was given the worst office, in an out-of-the-way location. I couldn't participate in our usual Friday evening drinks, because I had to get home to eat an early dinner instead. Those social contacts provided important work contacts as

well, and I really felt the impact of missing them.

If you continue to work while maintaining a high-risk pregnancy, it is essential for you to receive support and encouragement. You need to hear from colleagues and supervisors that they believe in your skills, that they understand your temporarily lowered productivity and know you will produce well again after the baby is born. But this kind of emotional backing is rare. Instead of getting credit for managing a difficult situation admirably by accommodating a high-risk pregnancy at work, your colleagues may insinuate that your work is simply not up to par.

Your boss's attitude in helping you adapt your work to a high-risk pregnancy can make a crucial difference. If your manager values your work and wants you to continue in your position after the baby's birth, you can work together to find an acceptable solution.

Ruth, who had previously lost a pregnancy in midterm, had a cervical cerclage and was on partial bed rest at home for much of the pregnancy that eventually produced her healthy daughter. With her boss's backing, Ruth discovered ways to manage working at home:

> My boss was very understanding, and he didn't want to lose me. I felt I was still part of something, and this way my mind was very busy and I didn't develop a negative attitude about the pregnancy.
>
> I work with computers, so I had a computer set up next to my bed. Most of my customers whom I dealt with by phone didn't know I had ever been out of the office.

If you are working during a high-risk pregnancy and do not have the support of your boss, try to find at least one colleague you trust so you have someone to talk to about the daily stresses you face. If this is impossible, try to reduce emotional stress during your pregnancy by talking with a friend or relative, or through the help of a pregnancy loss support group or sessions with a psychotherapist.

In spite of the impact pregnancy loss has on your career, you may discover that practical aspects of your struggle give you confidence to cope with your future. As one woman remarked, 'I think coping with my losses and managing difficult pregnancies have actually improved my ability to handle almost anything.'

What Can Help When Pregnancy Loss Affects Your Career

As a mother, you may find that your work is affected by your pregnancy loss. Whether you had planned a long or a short maternity leave, the idea of returning to the same place of employment after your loss, where you had been pregnant and looking forward to motherhood, can feel unbearable at first.

You may find solace in your work or in pursuing new professional challenges after a loss. On the other hand, you might discover that your job or professional training have temporarily lost meaning and importance and that your career has become an upsetting reminder of the absent baby.

If you face a high-risk pregnancy in the future, you must deal with putting your career second to your pregnancy or placing it completely on hold. You carry the double burden of uncertainty about future parenthood while being deprived of a full investment in your job. If you plan to return to your position, you will confront major logistical challenges as you arrange coverage for a pregnancy leave or alter your work routine to accommodate medical appointments and tests. And you may receive recognition from colleagues or managers for the difficulty of these tasks.

Making career decisions after a pregnancy loss, or in view of a future high-risk pregnancy, requires good social support to help sustain you until you begin to feel better again. Here are some additional suggestions:

- If you had planned a maternity leave, consider taking some of that time as a personal leave after your loss.
- Your job may be a welcome focus for your energies or may be an upsetting reminder of the absent baby. As grief resolves, your career can again provide a sense of purpose and become an important means of self-expression and source of self-esteem.
- If you are working during a high-risk pregnancy, consider talking to your boss about your special circumstances and the adjustments you will need to make in your work routine. Try to enlist his or her understanding and support.
- Try to find at least one supportive person at work whom you can talk to. If this isn't possible, look for emotional support outside work, with your family, friends, a pregnancy loss support group, or a counsellor. It

can help to know these people will be there for you whether or not
the pregnancy succeeds.

CHAPTER 15

PREGNANCY LOSS AND INFERTILITY: A TWOFOLD LOSS

W hen you experience both pregnancy loss and infertility – difficulty in conceiving and sustaining a pregnancy – you endure a double blow. Both pregnancy loss and infertility may deny you the number of biological children you want. They can turn the years in which you and your partner planned to have children and raise a family into an epoch of heartache and frustration. This double loss probably affects every aspect of your life, sometimes for years, as you withstand medical interventions and efforts to conceive, followed by hope and perhaps disappointment again.

Although infertility is usually defined as an inability to conceive after one year of unprotected sexual intercourse, other distinctions are made when it occurs in combination with pregnancy loss. Primary infertility, in which the woman has never conceived, can be followed by pregnancies that end in loss. Secondary infertility occurs when an inability to conceive follows a conception, whether the pregnancy ends in a loss or a birth. Included in this discussion are women who conceive but repeatedly lose pregnancies, usually within the first trimester, as they are unable to carry a pregnancy to term. One in six couples in the UK experience difficulties when trying to conceive.

Enduring the combined problem of pregnancy loss and infertility is particularly difficult because the period of hope, intervention, and frustration can continue for years. This lack of closure exacts an enormous price, as you remain in a prolonged state of limbo, with efforts to conceive and maintain a pregnancy dominating your life.

If your pregnancy loss was followed by an inability to conceive or keep a pregnancy, you may experience a profound sense of frustration and disbelief. After all, you were pregnant before. Why not again? In the case of newborn death followed by infertility, where you had a chance to parent your infant, however briefly, not having your own baby becomes a loss you can almost taste and feel. 'I think parental instincts are aroused when you hear *your* baby cry, see *your* baby, touch *your* baby,' explained one woman. 'For me, that brief experience of mothering has made my infertility more poignant, has given an edge to my frustration.'

If a couple does not have a subsequent, successful pregnancy, they may be grateful for having had the experience of carrying a baby, even for a short time. A woman's sense of herself and her femininity may seem more complete than if she had never been pregnant at all. Bess experienced three early losses before she was diagnosed as having premature ovarian failure:

> I am very sentimental about my pregnancies. I felt sick and horrible, but blooming with fruit. I'm so glad I experienced what it is like to be pregnant. I would have been very sorry to have missed it.

The experience of pregnancy loss is intensified if it comes after years of infertility. You may have felt you had conceived a 'miracle baby,' that your patience and persistence had finally been rewarded. To lose a baby after such major investments in time and effort can feel unspeakably unfair. You may also find you are already emotionally depleted from your infertility problems as you struggle to cope with the tragic outcome of our long-awaited pregnancy. 'We had spent six years of our lives in a futile quest that continued to bring us ever greater agony,' remarked one man whose wife finally conceived and carried a pregnancy to term, only to have their newborn infant die. 'We felt very betrayed by fate, as if we were under a cloud of doom.'

If you have a child and have also experienced pregnancy loss followed by secondary infertility, you face additional problems. You may feel cut off from most supportive people and informal networks, which are a lifeline for many infertile couples. Infertile couples without children have no sympathy for you, and parents who have the number of children they want may tell you that one child should be enough. They may even shun you, treating you as a failure.

But losses related to secondary infertility are very real. If you wanted at least two children, you must live with the disappointment that your family feels incomplete. You may have definite feelings about *not* wanting to raise an only child and may worry that you have cheated your offspring doubly, first by being emotionally unavailable during your efforts to conceive, and then by not providing a sibling. And after experiencing pregnancy loss and infertility, you can be left with a palpable sense of fear that your single child may come to some harm.

When to Stop Trying

People have different thresholds for the sadness of pregnancy loss and the rigours of fertility treatments. For some couples, it is very important not to give up. Others are ready sooner.

When prolonged efforts to conceive and maintain a pregnancy fail, your cumulative disappointment can be overwhelming. In addition to losing one or more pregnancies, you are deprived of your hoped-for future children who may never be born. One social worker with experience of infertility issues captures what these losses mean to would-be parents. 'A couple must actually mourn their pregnancy losses and infertility, grieving and "burying" their unborn, wished-for children,' she says. 'Only then can they be ready for other life-affirming possibilities, such as adoption or child-free living.'

It is important to decide at what point to stop trying for a biological child and take stock of your alternatives instead. This stopping point can be elusive, because continuing medical advances hold out new treatment possibilities and hope. Infertility specialists often feel their mission is to help you become pregnant, and rarely help you recognize when to stop trying. Even if you do stop, you may be haunted by the possibility that your next attempt might have succeeded.

Virginia had a healthy son followed by three miscarriages before she was diagnosed as having an antibody abnormality that resulted in her body rejecting her pregnancies. The efficacy of treatment was uncertain, but she was determined to try:

> If I give up, and never have a second child, then I'll have a feeling of failure forever. I hope I will have the good grace to know when I should stop, but at this point I need to keep trying.

Family and friends who fail to respect your personal timetable and motivation for continuing to try may urge you to abandon your hopes for a biological child. Rebecca, the mother of two adopted children, resented hearing others' opinions on how she and her husband should handle their decision:

> During the time we were so disappointed about not getting pregnant, friends and family would say, 'Why don't you look into adoption?' or

'Why don't you at least get on the adoption lists while you keep trying to have a baby?' But I was so hurt that they had given up on us when I wasn't ready to give up.

Discontinuing efforts to conceive when you desperately want a child can leave you feeling sad and defeated, especially since you have suffered pregnancy loss as well. 'I feel unfinished,' admitted the mother of one healthy child who had endured a late pregnancy loss and infertility treatments. 'My reproductive years have been long and I've been through a lot. But I want to feel the completion, the closure, and I don't.'

But continuing protracted and expensive attempts to conceive and hold on to a pregnancy can also exact a heavy toll, controlling all aspects of your life, from your sexual relationship to your personal finances. 'I am constantly thinking, What are my ovaries doing? What are the sperm doing?' one woman recalled. 'It makes it hard to enjoy anything else.'

At some point the treatments and relentless preoccupation with trying to conceive and maintain a pregnancy become worse than the problem, and the cost, both emotionally and financially, becomes too high to bear. A woman may be ready to stop treatment before her partner, partly because it often involves a regular invasion of her body and usually demands more of her time than his. Doctor's appointments might be taking precedence over all other commitments, including her career.

A woman may simply reach her limit, and decide to stop treatment for her own well being, even if her husband would like to keep trying. 'I couldn't bear it anymore,' one woman confessed. 'Mentally, I could not go on. I had to think of myself, to *save* myself, really.'

Partners sometimes reach the stopping point together, particularly if a medical risk arises. Sarah, who had suffered repeated early miscarriages, almost didn't come out of anaesthetic after her last D&C. The couple agreed that one more attempt would be their limit. As her husband said, 'I don't feel I have the right to risk her life with more pregnancies and would rather adopt instead.'

Occasionally a man may be ready to consider alternatives to pregnancy first. He may feel powerless over his wife's physical and emotional ordeal as he witnesses the monthly hope and anxiety when she ovulates and the inevitable depression when her menstrual period begins.

Philip and his wife developed infertility problems after a complicated delivery and newborn death. He found his willingness to consider adoption grew with their repeated, failed efforts to conceive:

I would like to have a child, but I do not want to have a child at all costs. Sometimes I think it would be better to adopt. It is hard to lie in bed and hear my wife crying because her period came. If there is something I can do to lessen what she is going through, I will do it.

A couple may find it easier to come to a joint decision about when to stop trying if they go together to as many medical appointments as possible. The man's presence and support can help the woman endure the demands placed on her and may enable him to empathize with her eventual weariness of the routine.

You may decide to stop trying as you see prime years passing you by, realizing you have given up other interests, or that you no longer enjoy yourself, one another, or your other children. For Sarah, the cumulative sacrifices she and her husband endured brought about a major transition:

Infertility and losses had been running my life. Getting pregnant was a problem. Holding on to the pregnancy was a problem. I want to have fun with my husband again. I want to talk about other things besides infertility tests and scans. We share so many other interests that we haven't enjoyed lately. I don't want this issue of having a baby to run our lives. My marriage is more important than just having a biological baby.

Having been pregnant before, you may find it difficult to give youself permission to stop your efforts to conceive, especially when medical advances can entice you to keep trying. When you do stop trying, you may feel as if you are quitting or failing.

One American infertility expert helps couples with this impasse by suggesting that a decision to stop does not make them 'quitters' or 'failures,' but instead is a constructive choice when the toll outweighs the likely benefits. The questions she has her clients ask themselves may help you to clarify your own readiness to make this choice:

- Do I know the likelihood of success? How can I find this out?
- What am I currently sacrificing to pursue this goal? How much am I willing to sacrifice?
- Are previously unacceptable options becoming more acceptable, such as adoption or child-free living?
- Would I feel a sense of relief if I skipped my next appointment with the infertility specialist or threw out the basal thermometer and

sperm collection jar?

- Have I just had enough? If it isn't time to stop, for me or for us, when will it be?

It takes a tremendous psychological leap to give up the dream of having a biological child. When you make this shift and are truly ready to stop trying, infertility and pregnancy losses will no longer define your existence. You might set new career goals, arrange special activities with an only child, take on a hobby, make exotic travel plans, or take steps to adopt a child. You may also experience renewed pleasure in your sexual relationship once you are released from the burden of sex on a timetable and obsessions about conceiving. A woman may feel particular relief once she is freed from the tyranny of the infertility and pregnancy-loss cycle. She can take pleasure in her body, exercising or losing weight for her own sake instead of preparing to carry a baby.

Once you have made your decision, you may also rediscover a refreshing capacity to empathize with other people who have different troubles. 'When you are going through infertility and losses, you feel like the most unfortunate person in the world,' explained Edna. 'When it's more resolved, you can again be sensitive to problems others may be having.'

Enduring Uncertainty

You may need to develop a number of coping strategies to help you endure the stress and uncertainties of both pregnancy loss and infertility. If you try to understand one another's depth of feeling, as well as your individual motivations to conceive, you can help each other and respect your mutual differences. 'I am willing to trust my wife's instincts about how important having a biological child is to her,' one husband explained. 'If she said three months are enough trying, I would trust that she knows what she needs to do.'

Husbands are often more optimistic about conceiving, while wives frequently remain tormented and anxious, making the kind of support each needs from the other very different. A wife usually wants her husband to listen to her worries, sympathize with her, and hug her. If he offers reassurances that ring false, or advice about what might solve the problem, he may genuinely mean well, but he runs the risk of leaving his partner even more angry and depressed than before.

Russell felt that undergoing a loss and infertility treatments had taught him a great deal about himself and the support his wife needed:

> I came with the attitude that this was a problem we could solve. I
> gradually realized I was incapable of solving it, that if it could be solved
> the doctors would do it. I needed to play a different role than fix-it
> man. I had to be supportive in a different way, to listen. And my wife
> learned to tell me what helped her.

Although it is important for a couple to communicate, it may also be
essential, at times, to limit discussions about infertility and losses.
Psychotherapist Merle Bombardieri proposes 'the twenty-minute rule,' in
which a couple sets a limit with a timer, between fifteen and thirty minutes
every day, for each partner to take turns venting current preoccupations.
After the timer goes off, no further discussion is allowed for that day. The
'rule' protects each partner from being overburdened by the other's turmoil,
yet encourages them to become aware of each other's concerns.

Both you and your partner may find outside support essential as you
grieve your losses and weather the uncertainties of infertility. Often this
support comes from others with similar problems, which can give you a
sense of community in your struggles. 'When I talk to my friends who are
also trying to become pregnant,' said one woman, 'I feel this incredible rush
of relief.'

Once you begin to put your troubles in perspective, you may feel more
stable and reassured. Instead of feeling mired in your disappointment, you
can eventually realize that you and your partner will have a future together,
no matter what. You may also feel confident you can make it a good future
even if unexpected adjustments are required. You may become aware that
your difficulties in having a family, while serious and prolonged, are among
the many challenges that couples encounter in marriage and in life. Other
families might not have this particular problem, but they still have their
share of misfortunes.

You may find the heartache of not having a biological child is
transformed over time with your capacity to grow and adapt to a difficult
reality. You can emerge with a feeling of inner strength, with humility,
wisdom, and a sense of humanity that are expressed in your dedication to
make the very most of the gifts life has given you. As Jessica expressed:

> What I have been through is a blessing in a very peculiar way. I always
> felt I would never be up to a major tragedy. I felt I would dissolve,
> shatter, not be capable of surviving a terrible loss. I find I am made out

of concrete. I have been changed. This has given me a good sense of myself.

Philip's view of becoming a parent, of his personal needs and goals, changed in significant ways after suffering a late pregnancy loss followed by infertility:

> Part of having a child is a selfish feeling, wanting to have a child for *me*, to make me feel good. There is also a feeling that I can *give* something to another person, teach them, raise them to be a good human being. Before we got pregnant our thoughts were more to have a child for us. Now we tend to think more of having a child to give to, a feeling that we can contribute something.

What Can Help You Cope with Pregnancy Loss and Infertility

The cumulative impact of pregnancy loss and infertility is immense. You have endured heartache, frustration, and anxiety-ridden pregnancies, sometimes over a period of years. In addition, you probably had to make major adjustments in your personal and professional goals. Your career and finances may have revolved around infertility treatments or attempts to maintain precarious pregnancies for a long time.

In addition to the financial drain, you are probably paying a high price in time and emotions as efforts to conceive take over your life, leaving little energy or interest for either your relationship or other pursuits. This combination of problems is particularly heartbreaking as you struggle to make the best decision about treatments and when to stop trying to conceive, either accepting the number of children you have or considering alternatives to pregnancy.

Here are some suggestions to help you endure the combined stresses of pregnancy loss and infertility:

- Respect your need to grieve each pregnancy loss before embarking on intensive infertility treatments.
- If you suspect an infertility problem, or have had two consecutive early miscarriages, consider seeing a reproductive endocrinologist for a complete medical evaluation and possible treatment.

- For women, you might suggest that your partner go to doctors' appointments with you, both for support and to increase mutual understanding of the strain involved. Try following 'the twenty-minute rule,' in which each of you takes twenty minutes daily to unburden feelings about your losses or treatment. This can help you keep communication open but prevent you becoming overburdened with the other's concerns.

- Try to find outside support. No one experiencing both pregnancy loss and infertility should have to go through this ordeal alone. If you know friends with similar problems, see if you can support one another. Consider contacting your local branch of ISSUE, or arranging to see a psychotherapist.

- Well-chosen reading material that keeps you up-to-date on diagnostic and treatment options can be very useful. There are also excellent books available on alternatives to having a pregnancy and the experiences of other couples who have chosen different solutions, such as adoption or child-free living. See Appendix D for some suggestions.

- Try to get involved with outside interests. Pregnancy loss and infertility treatments can become all-consuming. Other activities can be a welcome distraction and can also help you discover creative outlets and develop potential in other areas.

- It is important to examine honestly your feelings about your losses and infertility treatment, the toll they take, and your motivation to keep trying for a successful pregnancy. Share your appraisal frankly with your partner, so you can make decisions based on understanding and respect for each other. Know that it takes courage to continue trying to conceive but that it also takes courage and wisdom to know when to stop and direct your energies elsewhere.

CHAPTER 16

BECOMING PREGNANT AGAIN

The biggest negative impact of my losses has been that each subsequent pregnancy is a fearful time instead of a happy time for me. I wish I could have that innocent feeling, that I could fly through pregnancy not realizing the risks. I am envious of women in that position. They are having such an easy, joyous time!

JULIA

A pregnancy that follows a loss can be fraught with anxiety and ambivalence. A subsequent pregnancy is usually not the carefree, joyous experience you may have had the first time you expected a baby. You probably want desperately to feel elation, but you are too apprehensive to relish the miracle of your pregnancy.

Enduring a loss may affect your decision to conceive again, your perception of carrying the new baby, and your experience of giving birth. It can have an impact on your relationship to your partner and on the way you raise your children. Understanding and accepting how your life has been altered can help you make decisions about future pregnancies and childrearing that are right for you.

Making the Decision

Like most parents, you probably experience a healthy amount of ambivalence during any pregnancy. You may wonder what impact a first child will have on your life or how your other children will react to a new baby. Losing a pregnancy may strengthen your commitment, encouraging you to discard any hesitancy and forge ahead with plans to conceive again quickly. On the other hand, the experience could leave you so doubtful of success, and fearful of experiencing another loss, that you avoid resolving the issue for months.

Researchers have discovered that if parents conceive too soon after a loss they may be unable to express their grief, delaying and complicating their emotional recovery. Women in particular fare better emotionally if they wait at least six months before conceiving again. Grieving your baby's loss is an absorbing process that may interfere with your ability to bond with your new child. If you fail to acknowledge and accept the loss before trying to have another child, you can fall into the trap of hoping to replace the baby you carried and lost. You may also become unduly fearful during the next pregnancy.

Michael and Judi Forman, who wrote about the loss of their newborn son in an article for a parenting magazine, explained how important a grieving period was to them:

> Before we could open ourselves up to the possibility of having another child, we needed to reach some understanding of *why* Robin died, what his death meant to us in terms ranging from the most concrete to the most spiritual. Without that awareness it is unlikely that we could have become loving or effective parents to another baby.

The Right Timing

When a couple decides to conceive again depends on the kind of loss they suffered, the mother's age, and each parent's emotional timetable. Doctors generally recommend that a couple wait two or three full menstrual cycles before trying to conceive again following any loss. This passage of time not only allows for emotional recovery to begin but also permits the uterus to return to its normal size, the lining to grow back, and the cervix to close, all of which might improve the chances of success in a subsequent pregnancy.

But a doctor's clear-cut medical permission to try again does not take into account all the issues a bereaved couple must weigh. Lisa had lost a newborn daughter and felt nervous about conceiving again. Even after the requisite three-month period had passed, she fretted over being physically and emotionally ready:

> When my husband and I started discussing getting pregnant again, I was very hesitant about sex or even trying to conceive at first. On one hand, I said, 'Yes, I want another baby,' and on the other I said, 'No, I'm too nervous, scared, and confused.'

Some parents are afraid that if they conceive again quickly, they will be too vulnerable if they suffer a subsequent loss. Others feel surprisingly relaxed about trying to conceive again. One mother had been panicky about conceiving her first pregnancy, which ended with the death of her newborn baby. Keeping track of temperature charts and fertile periods had taken its toll before the first conception, so when she and her husband agreed to become pregnant after their loss, the pressure was off:

> I at least knew I had been pregnant before, so I was much more relaxed. The fact that I felt I wasn't quite ready also made me a lot less anxious about conceiving. If it happened, it happened. If it didn't happen right away, that was okay, too.

Older mothers may feel more pressure to conceive quickly after a loss because they realize their best childbearing years are rapidly diminishing. They run the risk of forging ahead with little consideration of their emotional recovery and physical readiness because they feel the time constraint so keenly. 'Waiting was the hardest,' one thirty-six-year-old woman recalled. 'I wanted to fast-forward my life so I could just start trying to get pregnant again.'

Young women may find they are not immune to feeling similar pressures, even if they have many good childbearing years ahead of them. Karen had experienced several first-trimester losses while in her twenties and found that with each disappointment, the urgency to conceive again increased. 'I feel I've got to make up for all the losses and the lost time,' she admitted. 'It's an indescribably urgent feeling.'

If you and your partner's timetables for conceiving again are not aligned, try to discuss your conflicts openly and honestly until both of you are closer to an agreement. You will need each other's emotional support during your next pregnancy, especially if it will be high-risk, so it is important to wait until both of you are truly ready.

Once you have agreed to conceive again, you may find that every aspect of your life is refracted through the prism of planning a subsequent pregnancy. 'My husband and I had to plot out his business trips to coincide with my fertile periods,' remarked one woman, 'and then we had to make sure he was around during the critical first trimester, when I usually miscarried. It placed a tremendous strain on both of us.'

It is difficult to anticipate all the issues and to predict the best time to conceive, but being honest with yourself, your partner, and your doctor about your feelings can help you arrive at an acceptable decision.

Finding Out You Are Pregnant Again

Once you have decided to conceive again, you await the arrival of each menstrual period with mixed emotions, cautiously hopeful and yet fearing another loss. Confirmation of a new pregnancy brings hope for a happy outcome, but it also can begin months of anxiety as you wait for the birth of your new child. This pregnancy may remind you of your loss more than you had anticipated, especially when you reach the point at which you lost the previous baby.

Some parents are reluctant to believe in the pregnancy or its outcome, refusing even to fantasize about the baby. Natalie, who suffered several first-trimester miscarriages, felt that by not allowing herself to commit her hopes to each pregnancy, she might be more prepared to handle a possible loss. 'Because of the miscarriages,' she confessed, 'I was not entirely invested in each of the subsequent pregnancies.'

Additional stresses can be placed on a marriage once the new pregnancy is confirmed if one or both partners are reluctant to have sexual relations. Doctors may advise a limit on sexual relations during a subsequent, high-risk pregnancy for several reasons. Uterine contractions associated with female orgasms, and certain components in semen, such as prostaglandins, have been implicated in the onset of premature labour.

Other stresses can emerge because the woman may be feeling vulnerable in her newly pregnant state and may make more demands on her partner's time and attention than usual. Even if she had been an independent, confident woman before her first loss, she can feel insecure and defenseless during a subsequent pregnancy.

Neil, whose wife had lost three pregnancies in the first trimester, at first welcomed the time-consuming nature of his career once their new pregnancy was confirmed. He was grateful for the haven from anxieties his work provided, but his wife felt he wasn't spending enough time with her or giving her the support she needed. When she called Neil at his office one day, he suddenly realized why he needed to change his attitude:

> I said I was busy and couldn't talk to her. I didn't even take the time to find out what was bothering her. It turned out she was staining and was very frightened. Whenever she called me after that incident, I always asked if it was important. If she said 'Yes,' I just dropped whatever I was doing and talked to her.

Once you have adjusted to the new pregnancy and the anxiety it provokes, you may be able to achieve a certain closeness to your partner by sharing your concerns for each other and the pregnancy. Neil eventually found a new role for himself that felt comfortable and important:

> Once I accepted that Sarah required extra help during this pregnancy, I found I had a tolerance for her needs and anxieties that wasn't there before. It was good knowing I was needed and that we could be there for each other.

The decisions and stresses you face once you have conceived again begin to multiply as the pregnancy advances. You wonder when to tell other people about the pregnancy and question if you are receiving the right medical care. Perhaps most difficult of all, you begin the endless weeks of anxiety, hoping against hope, but never quite believing, that all will go well.

Telling Others

The joy you felt with your first pregnancy may have intensified as you shared your good news with family and friends. In a pregnancy following a loss, this eagerness often becomes stifled, replaced with a sense of caution and privacy. 'We held off telling even immediate family until the beginning of the third month,' explained Neil. 'I couldn't go screaming to the world about how happy I was with the pregnancy. I couldn't enjoy it with other friends and family the way I would have liked to.'

Keeping the pregnancy a secret becomes a way of trying to contain the tension and stanch the flow of sorrow if another loss occurs. This is partly because sharing the news about the pregnancy can mean spreading anxiety and concern among loved ones you wish to spare.

But this caution can also backfire because it deprives you of a support network of family and friends during this anxious time – and in the event of another loss. Ellen and her husband had agreed to wait to announce their subsequent pregnancy until after the results of the amniocentesis were available, well into the fifth month of pregnancy. But by the time she had reached twelve weeks. Ellen had changed her mind. 'I felt I needed more support from everyone around me by then,' she recalled, 'so my husband and I talked it over again and we agreed to start telling at least close friends and family that week.'

Not everyone you tell about the new pregnancy will necessarily respond with joy and elation. They may be so personally concerned or professionally dubious that they cannot be encouraging. Gail and her husband experienced two full-term losses of babies with rare congenital anomalies and had to change doctors to find one who would support their efforts to try again.

The few people who knew Gail and her husband were trying to conceive again thought they were being irresponsible, including her parents. 'But it was impossible to get cross with my parents,' she conceded, 'because they basically were just so worried and anxious about me and my husband. My father couldn't even talk about the new pregnancy, not even after our healthy son was born.'

A different problem can occur when relatives and friends who were supportive at first lose patience with your continuing anxiety once the pregnancy is progressing nicely. They do not understand how much is riding on the pregnancy or how fearful you are about the outcome. Annette, who had suffered infertility problems and a miscarriage, felt criticized by friends for her ongoing concern and even began to fault herself for her worries:

> All the anxieties overrode the joy, and I started to berate myself for that. But I feel I was wrong to berate myself. It is natural to feel anxious after a loss, and I should have been kinder to myself.

Some people may even tell the pregnant mother that worrying during a subsequent pregnancy could cause another loss or produce a high-strung baby. As one woman who received such comments said:

> These remarks were not only cruel but also unfounded. After two miscarriages, all I could do was worry during my next pregnancy. But from the day we brought our healthy son home from the hospital, he slept through the night. He was a relaxed, happy baby in spite of all my anxieties while pregnant.

If a Loss Occurs Again

After the second loss, I fell apart. I had no self-esteem. I kept thinking, 'Everyone can do this and I can't. This is going to keep happening.' I didn't know if I could keep trying and having more losses.

AMY

With a subsequent conception, most couples face the same one-in-five chance of losing a baby as the rest of the population; however, if they suffer more than one pregnancy loss, they may begin to feel like a statistical oddity. 'It was as if lightning had indeed struck twice,' lamented one mother. 'We felt we had been singled out in some awful way.'

The most important step you can take at this point is to seek thorough and thoughtful medical care to optimize your chances for a healthy future pregnancy. Exploring the physical causes and treatments for your loss can help your frame of mind as well, enabling you to take meaningful action when your life feels so out of control. 'The more we learned and the more we understood,' recalled Neil, 'the easier it became for us to cope with our situation.'

When you and your partner schedule a consultation with your doctor, plan for the meeting by discussing and writing down your questions beforehand. If you still feel your questions are not being answered, consider changing doctors or at least obtaining a second opinion from a medical specialist.

When a subsequent pregnancy ends in another loss, you and your partner may need time off to rethink and re-establish your lives and priorities. Psychotherapy or a group like SANDS may be especially helpful. A group in particular can console you and enable you to reach out to others when you thought you had nothing left to give.

After her third loss, Neil's wife became a lay counsellor for couples who had suffered pregnancy losses. 'I think she basically integrated her sorrow into something positive,' recognized Neil, 'by trying to do something meaningful for others.'

Reconsidering Your Medical Care

A pregnancy loss may force you to re-evaluate your choice of doctors and the management of your medical care during your next pregnancy. In some instances, the loss itself may have created high-risk complications that require more specialized care for any subsequent pregnancy. If you stay with the same doctor, you may need more technological monitoring and additional interventions during your next pregnancy, and it is almost inevitable that you will be assigned to the care of a specialist.

You may be so upset by your loss that you and your partner feel compelled to switch doctors, even if you thought your original doctor was medically competent. You may be dissatisfied with the lack of comfort your doctor provided, or may feel that returning to the same doctor could make memories of your loss too painful. Seeking the care of a new, well-qualified doctor can bring a feeling of fresh hope for your next pregnancy.

Changing Doctors

*I*f you decide to change doctors for a subsequent pregnancy, there are several issues to bear in mind. Try to get solid recommendations from other patients and doctors, make an appointment with the prospective doctor, and ask pertinent questions that will reveal his attitude about pregnancy loss and your particular case. You may want to write down your questions and your medical history before the appointment, so you and your doctor can refer to this information. If he rushes you through your questions and dismisses your concerns, he is probably not the right doctor for you.

'I refused to go to one specialist who told me in the consultation not to worry, that I would have a baby,' said one woman who had experienced several miscarriages. 'I knew enough to realize that wasn't necessarily true and worried that his attitude would be all wrong for me.'

Keep in mind that highly skilled doctors do not necessarily have the best bedside manner. Both your doctor's competence and your feeling of being in a partnership with him are vital. During your consultation, ask the doctor if you may call for reassurances or come into the hospital without an appointment so that a midwife can let you hear the baby's heartbeat. If the answer is 'No' and you live in a large enough city to find another doctor, consider doing so.

When Molly changed doctors after her baby son was stillborn, she knew she would be extremely anxious throughout her next pregnancy and questioned her new obstetrician about his availability. 'He made it clear that if I needed to, I could come in anytime I wanted,' she recalled. 'He told me if I needed to see that the baby was alive on a particular day, all I had to do was turn up.'

Discussing all options and making the patient a part of the decision-making process can also help dispel a feeling of helplessness. Julia had several first-trimester miscarriages before she switched to a fetal medicine specialist in a large teaching hospital. He supported her quest for information and worked closely with her throughout her subsequent pregnancy, which resulted in the birth of a healthy daughter. 'We discussed everything,' she recalled, 'from how much Clomid I should take to what dosage of progesterone I should have. I felt this doctor was in partnership with me.'

Use of Technology

You may want your doctor to examine you more frequently and make greater use of available technology in a subsequent pregnancy. Although antenatal testing may be either reassuring or anxiety-provoking, the knowledge technology provides can be encouraging following a loss. 'I didn't have testing in my first pregnancy because I was so young,' explained Lisa, who was nervous after her full-term baby died from a congenital disorder, 'but I had three ultrasound scans in my next pregnancy. It was very encouraging to know the new baby was developing properly.'

You may find it especially reassuring to be under the care of a doctor who has testing and monitoring available but who evaluates your individual situation and discusses it with you and your partner, so you can decide together which procedures are useful and necessary. Weighing the risks and benefits of tests in a subsequent pregnancy becomes agonizing if your loss may have been triggered by a medical procedure. If you have concerns about specific tests, be prepared to take the initiative in bringing them up with your physician.

Paula and her doctor suspected that she lost her second pregnancy in midterm because her uterus did not tolerate an amniocentesis of a malformation. Even though she had since slipped into a higher-risk age group, she was reluctant to have the procedure in her next pregnancy. When her doctor assumed Paula would opt for amniocentesis because of her age, she confronted him:

> I forced the issue and said to him, 'I can't sleep at night thinking about having an amniocentesis. Let's just sit down and go through the pregnancy I lost and see if this could have been caused by the amniocentesis.' We went over everything and he finally said, 'You're right. I've been nervous about it, too.' I felt it was important to talk about not just the probabilities in amniocentesis, but about my particular case.

Even if your next baby is at risk for genetic or chromosomal abnormalities, you may decide against having a procedure because it presumes a willingness to abort an impaired pregnancy. 'It seemed inconceivable to have an abortion at twenty weeks if the amniocentesis revealed a problem,' recalled Lydia, who had suffered two losses and was thirty-six at the time of her subsequent pregnancy. She also recognized that the likelihood of genetic problems occurring was slightly less than the chance of losing the baby from the procedure itself. After talking it over with her husband and her doctor, Lydia decided against having amniocentesis.

These decisions can shift, however, in subsequent pregnancies. When Lydia found herself pregnant again at age forty, she recognized that both her chances of producing a defective baby and her inability to cope with a handicapped child had increased significantly. 'We were still reluctant to use amniocentesis because it is done so late in the pregnancy,' she concluded, 'so we opted for chorionic villus sampling, which is performed much earlier.'

If you decide to have antenatal tests that also reveal the baby's sex, consider having your doctor give you the information in a sealed envelope so you may carefully weigh the impact this news might have on you. Some parents believe that knowing the gender will enable them to bond with their new baby and think about their expected child as an individual. Others feel that knowing the sex of the new baby would make them sad, as they would compare this pregnancy to the one they lost. Try to do what feels best, and realize that your decision about having this information may change with later pregnancies.

Your involvement in medical care as a couple can also change following a loss. You and your partner may want to attend antenatal visits together, as your joint participation in the progress of the pregnancy can help you support each other during these stressful months. 'Going to doctor's appointments together during the next pregnancy helped us enormously after the stillbirth,' one woman said. 'It enabled us to keep communication open about sexual relations and what tests to have, really all the issues that affected us as a couple.'

Whatever our decisions may be – to stay with your current doctor or to change doctors, to use more technology or less – you may find that you change your mind and readjust your thinking during the pregnancy. Try not to be embarrassed about asking for different care from your doctor or about finding a more expert and compassionate doctor. A good practitioner will make every effort to ensure you have the best treatment available, even if he can't provide it.

Surviving the New Pregnancy

I felt I was walking on eggs and just kept hoping this time it would be okay.   STELLA

When you conceive after one or more losses, the new pregnancy can create immense hopes, anxieties, and unexpected conflicts. You may be unable to concentrate at work or to enjoy leisure activities. If you have other children, you may discover that they give you great satisfaction and provide welcome distractions from your anxious state. When you are trying to concentrate on the new pregnancy, however, you may sometimes resent their intrusions. If they are old enough to know about your loss and the new pregnancy, they may increase your anxiety by asking in all innocence, 'Will this baby die, too?'

This continuous worry may keep you from bonding readily to the expected baby for fear of suffering another loss. On the other hand, a mother in particular may become devoted both quickly and intensely, believing that if the pregnancy fails, she will have experienced her unborn baby as much as possible. 'I want to bond immediately with this baby, because if it doesn't work out, I want to enjoy it as much as I can,' one woman explained. 'I like to think this baby senses that commitment, too, and wants to stay with me.'

This special subsequent pregnancy can become a dominant concern in the expectant mother's life. Some women practically memorize pregnancy books, carefully following every suggestion, or curtail activities even beyond what their doctors recommend. Others debate whether to stop work or forgo regular exercise routines, and let their partners, relatives, or friends take over meal preparation and housework.

A woman may even keep herself housebound because she feels this protects the pregnancy. Julia had experienced three miscarriages, but when she became pregnant again she chose to keep herself housebound because she believed that as long as she stayed home, she would be fine. 'I felt very fragile,' she admitted. 'I feared going out of the house to the point where I felt I was becoming phobic.'

During a subsequent pregnancy, you and your partner may become overly cautious about making plans for the new baby. The layette you eagerly set up during the previous pregnancy may stay hidden away until the baby is safely born. You may put away gifts unopened, and not discuss names for the new infant until your baby arrives. If avoiding preparations for the baby helps you survive the new pregnancy, respect your feelings. You can ask a friend or relative to shop right after the baby is born or set up the cot in time for your homecoming.

Some expectant mothers and fathers find their approaches to coping with a subsequent pregnancy are at odds. Neil attempted to find strength within himself during their most recent pregnancy. 'I didn't have much difficulty with the lack of assurances during this last pregnancy,' he declared after his wife safely carried to term following several miscarriages. 'I had faith, not that the pregnancy would work out, which it did, but that if it didn't work out, I would be able to deal with it.'

But this feeling of strength was in stark contrast to his wife's experience, as she envisioned a variety of ways a loss could happen again. 'As a result,' Neil confessed, 'my wife felt more prepared for problems than I did, but she also lived in a constant state of upset because there was always that fear that something could go wrong.'

If you suffered an early loss, your new pregnancy may be fraught with both dread and optimism as each day passes without a problem. These mixed emotions intensify as the point of your previous loss arrives and then passes. As the baby continues to grow and you receive good antenatal test results, you may feel increasingly hopeful and confident that the pregnancy is advancing properly and that your baby will be fine.

Eric felt that his concern disappeared rapidly once he heard the heartbeat and saw the baby on the ultrasound screen. 'I felt the pregnancy was on its way, that it was really going to happen,' he admitted. Other parents find their sense of security peaks later, around the seventh month, the point at which the baby has a good chance of surviving outside the womb.

If you endured a late loss, no time in the pregnancy may ever seem safe, and your anxiety can increase as the due date approaches. Adam, who lost a full-term baby shortly after birth, remembered how anxious his wife became in her subsequent pregnancy. 'She waited and waited until the baby was big enough to feel his kicks,' he recalled. 'But then if the baby didn't kick for half a day, she would go crazy.'

Until particular medical or psychological hurdles have been passed, bereaved parents often try to assuage their anxiety by doing anything in their power to give their subsequent pregnancy its best chance. One mother used meditation tapes to help her go to sleep every night for three months until she got beyond her critical first trimester. Some expectant parents pray daily or bargain with God, pledging, 'If you give me this baby, I'll do anything you want!'

Otherwise rational and scientifically minded people have been known to seek out faith healers or mystics and to wear charms that are supposed to help maintain a pregnancy. Old wives' tales are revived and ancient customs dusted off in an attempt to defy the fates – or at least lessen anxiety – during the months of waiting and worrying.

Parents may freely admit that submitting to such talismans is like believing in voodoo, but they adhere to the customs steadfastly. Karen felt that visiting a religious faith healer was only part of the total process of trying to secure her subsequent pregnancy. 'I felt we were seeing all these doctors and using medical interventions,' she said, 'and this didn't seem all that different to me.' When the healer suggested she wear a magnet around her neck throughout the pregnancy, citing ancient biblical references to lodestones, Karen eagerly complied. 'I've been wearing one around my neck under my shirt since I found out I was pregnant,' she conceded. 'I worry about someone noticing it and having to explain it, but I wear it all the time.'

Endurance may come from unexpected sources. A sense of humour can be the key to surviving a pregnancy after a loss. 'What is life without being able to laugh at it?' one woman asserted. 'I try to suppress my very satirical side most of the time, but I let it out when I'm pregnant. It really helps me deal with the stress.' Keeping a diary can be a wonderful outlet for your worries during a stressful pregnancy. 'Whenever I had trouble coping,' explained Molly, 'I opened my diary and wrote down my thoughts.'

As you approach the new baby's due date, you may wish to take a parentcraft course but can't bear the thought of being in a roomful of expectant couples who have never experienced a loss. Consider arranging private lessons for yourself and your partner through the NCT. You may also want to ask your doctor if you may have a supportive professional, with you at the birth, in addition to your partner.

No matter what kind of loss you suffered, you will probably need to hear the cry of your healthy newborn, and see for yourself that she is strong and well, before you begin to relax and enjoy your baby and parenthood.

For Mothers Who Must Manage a Subsequent High-Risk Pregnancy

If you are a mother who has experienced a medical crisis in a previous pregnancy, such as premature labour or high blood pressure, your subsequent conceptions may require additional interventions and vigilance. The increased doctor's visits and monitoring for a high-risk pregnancy may elevate your anxieties, affecting your relationships at home or your productivity at work. The overpowering impact this can have on your work life is discussed in Chapter 14, 'The Impact of Pregnancy Loss on Your Career.'

Bed rest is perhaps the most trying intervention required by some high-risk pregnancies. Women who must stay on complete bed rest may find it hard to be in a totally dependent state, whether at home or in the hospital. Nicole, an active and self-reliant woman, was in need of constant care during her pregnancies because of recurrent premature labour. She couldn't afford professional home care, but having her mother-in-law come to help was not a problem-free solution, either:

> Having someone who has always seen you as independent is a little embarrassing. It's hard to keep bothering a family member to get you lunch or something to drink. As willing as my mother-in-law was, I felt uncomfortable constantly asking her for things.

Although you are physically dependent, you can still find ways to exert some control. If you are at home with a relative, or hospitalized with professionals caring for you, make an effort to assert your needs. One hospitalized woman described feeling guilty about asking for nursing help in getting her dirty dishes cleared away. Yet the atmosphere in her ward was important for her morale, so she overcame her reluctance to be demanding. You, too, will probably feel better if you act on the choices you do have.

After one midterm loss and a threatened miscarriage, Amelia was put on home bed rest for her next pregnancy. The complicated, long-range planning her situation demanded actually helped Amelia feel she was exercising some control. She matched people who were willing to help with the tasks that needed to be done:

> My sister and friends who enjoy cooking just loved creating meals for me and putting calories on someone else. Deciding what needed to be done and who could do it best was a benefit to the people who wanted to help as well as to me.

If you have a young child, managing bed rest at home becomes even more of a challenge. It is frustrating when your child wants to play or gets into things she shouldn't and you aren't supposed to get up and chase her. Make an effort to arrange adequate child care so you don't have to choose between caring for your youngster or your unborn baby.

Surviving the loneliness and isolation of bed rest, especially in a hospital, can be agonizing. You may find that bringing bed linen from home lifts your spirits during the weeks or months of your hospitalized pregnancy. 'Wearing my own brightly coloured T-shirts helped me feel better about myself,' one woman asserted. 'So did putting on earrings and a little makeup each morning.'

It may be especially helpful to give some structure to your day by waking up at a certain time, bathing at a certain time, and having a specific period set aside for projects. Try making appointments with friends and family who want to see you, so you avoid having too many visitors at once or none at all when you really want the company. This also prevents someone from walking in when you are having a sponge bath.

See if you can think of innovative ways to keep occupied. Needlepoint, knitting, or other crafts can keep your hands and mind engaged. You might even arrange for tutouring on a topic that is especially enjoyable and interesting to you. 'I had always wanted to brush up on my French,' remembered Amelia, 'but I never had time. So that was one of the first things I planned when I knew most of my next pregnancy would be spent in the hospital.'

For women who need to be hospitalized at a medical facility far from their homes, the feeling of seclusion only increases, and the courage and effort needed to cope can become monumental. Marianne suffered from an incompetent cervix and was hospitalized for several months in a teaching hospital about an hour and half from her home. Her husband endured the journey three times a week and stayed with friends near the hospital at weekends. She received wonderful support from friends and colleagues who visited her, sent notes, and called. 'There wasn't a spot on the wall that wasn't covered by cards,' she recalled.

Extended bed rest can make you feel that your body and muscle tone have been impaired, drastically affecting your self-image. 'I could barely walk after my son was delivered at thirty weeks,' said Amelia, who spent most of the pregnancy in the hospital. 'I hadn't gained weight so much, but it was as if my leg muscles had collapsed and slipped down around my ankles. As thrilled as I was about my baby's birth, I felt and looked terrible.'

If you are a new mother who has just come off bed rest, try to be patient with yourself and your physical condition, since it will take time for you to feel back in shape. For every week in bed you will need about three weeks to regain your former condition. Talk with your doctor, nurse, or physiotherapist about exercises to do daily that will gradually increase your strength and muscle tone.

Parenting After Your Loss

Once you and your partner deliver a healthy baby, the vestiges of your loss may continue to colour your experiences of parenthood. From the moment of birth through your child's first illness, you may find yourself plagued by more anxieties than other parents. Even red-letter events occurring years later, such as your child's first day of school or first night away from home, can bring back recollections of uneasiness related to your pregnancy loss. Understanding the source of your concerns can help you overcome them and allow your living children to emerge from the shadow of your sorrow.

Experiencing the Birth of a Healthy Baby

The delivery of a healthy baby may be highly emotional, as memories of your previous pregnancy crowd your mind. Thoughts of your earlier pregnancy may upset you or may be a bittersweet reminder of the baby you lost.

When Molly gave birth to her daughter, she found she needed to think about her stillborn son, in spite of remarks she felt were intended to deflect her thoughts away from him. 'People tried to say such uplifting things about the new baby as 'She's so healthy,' but all I could think was, "Now I know what we were missing with our son."'

The birth experience itself may trigger thoughts of concern that had been repressed while you coped with the new pregnancy. Because of her past history and loss, Paula had a caesarean delivery, which proceeded in a very orderly fashion. 'But when our son emerged alive and healthy, my whole body suddenly shook with this enormous sigh of relief,' she recalled. 'I hadn't realized how tense I had been during the entire pregnancy until my son was born and I knew he was fine.'

Even normal experiences following the birth of a healthy child can be highly charged. Many parents realize that not all babies cry instantly at birth, but mothers and fathers who have suffered a pregnancy loss may feel panic-stricken when they don't hear their babies cry as soon as they are born. '"Why isn't my baby crying? Do something!"' Lisa recalled yelling at the delivery room staff when her healthy son was born. 'When he finally cried I felt enormous relief.'

Even hearing your healthy baby's cry may not immediately dispel the fear of possibly losing another child. 'I couldn't believe she was alive,' Molly admitted. 'I had been so afraid to hope, I didn't allow myself the thought that she would live, even when I heard her cry.'

This disbelief in your baby's safe arrival is not an unusual reaction after a loss. You may need to grieve the baby who died once again as you gradually realize that this new, different baby is going to be strong and well.

Problems with Childrearing

The effects of your pregnancy loss can persist long after your new baby is safely delivered. Disciplining long-awaited children can be a problem after the many disappointments you have endured along the way to becoming a parent. You may find yourself reluctant to reprimand your children properly, even when you know the youngsters need constraints. One mother conceded that her son became hopelessly spoiled because of her fears. 'But once I realized that discipline could be an act of love, that I could make my child adapt better to the world around him if he learned what some of the limits were,' she confessed, 'we both did much better.'

You may also feel protective of your children's health and welfare, running to the GP sooner than parents who haven't had losses. 'I still get nervous whenever my son gets ill,' acknowledged one mother. 'I know I overreact and am a little obsessed.'

If vigilant medical care for your baby gives you peace of mind, you are entitled to those precautionary doctors' visits. Explain your concerns to your GP and consider arranging telephone consultations to determine when your child needs to be seen. Your feelings of panic when your child gets ill should diminish as he grows.

Pregnancy loss, and the poignant recognition of how fleeting life is, can leave you a positive legacy as a parent as well. 'I'm more patient with our son than I think I would have been if we had not lost our daughter the year before,' concluded Paul. 'I guess I'm just mindful of his preciousness even when he is driving me mad.'

Responding to Awkward Questions

As your subsequent pregnancy advances and after the new baby is born, you might receive unintentionally provocative comments from well-wishers who ask, 'Is this your first baby?' or 'How many other children do you have?'

Molly, who suffered a full-term stillbirth, had difficulty responding to these questions after her healthy daughter was born. Sometimes she would just say that her daughter wasn't her first child and leave it at that, without saying anything more unless people asked further questions. Some did. If they persisted, she would say something simple, such as 'My son died.' For Molly, these answers became another way of establishing her son's existence. 'He *was* real,' she asserted, 'even more so after our daughter was born.'

How you decide to handle these questions is very individual. Talk over your feelings with your partner, and try to answer depending on how well you know each person and what feels most comfortable. You may choose to say you had a baby who died, or you may prefer not to tell strangers or acquaintances of your loss. Not mentioning the baby to others does not mean you have forgotten your child.

Understand that your answer may change with time, as your family grows and the loss becomes less painful. You may struggle with feelings of guilt at first, because you are not always publicly acknowledging the baby who died, but eventually you will come to a private peace about your relationship to that child. Lisa had lost a daughter and then had a healthy son, whom she sometimes told people was her first child. She recalled, however, saying to herself, 'Lucy we haven't forgotten about you; we still love you.'

What Can Help You Survive a Subsequent Pregnancy

Pregnancy after a loss can be a roller coaster of joy and anxiety. Just making the decision to conceive again might throw you and your partner into a state of apprehension. Once you have agreed to try again, you may face new worries about medical treatments and the concern that the outcome of any subsequent pregnancy could be equally uncertain.

When you have conceived after a loss, you must resolve how and when you tell other people about your pregnancy. Even the experiences of giving birth to a healthy child and taking her home to raise can be coloured by your loss.

Here are some suggestions that may help ease you through the tensions of a subsequent pregnancy and the tumultuous feelings it will inevitably produce:

- Try to keep in mind that emotional readiness and physical readiness to conceive again are not always in synch, nor do partners always agree on when to become pregnant again. Make an effort to be as open and honest about your readiness as you can.
- When you conceive again, plan on whom you will tell and when you will tell them about the new pregnancy. Try to keep your own comfort uppermost in your mind.
- Accept your need to take charge of certain aspects of your next pregnancy. Consider working out a plan to have access to your doctor and your specialist if you feel this will give your subsequent pregnancy the best chance of succeeding.
- Even with the best possible medical care and emotional support, you may still feel anxious at times. This is understandable, so try to be patient with yourself.
- If your subsequent pregnancy ends in another loss, give yourself time to grieve, then consider involvement in activities that may bring you comfort and that will honour your baby.
- As the expectant mother, if you are bedridden during your pregnancy, respect your need to exert control when you can. Consider creating a schedule, and make your environment as pleasant as possible. Find projects to keep you busy, and try not to be embarrassed about asking for what you need.
- When well-meaning people ask you and your partner how many children you have, find a response that is comfortable for you at the moment, understanding that it may shift with time as you integrate your loss into your life.

MANAGING PROBLEM PREGNANCIES

Once a diagnosis of a problem has been made, there are a variety of approaches to treating specific kinds of threatened pregnancy loss and preparing for a subsequent high-risk pregnancy. Some tests and procedures are well-accepted practices that are readily available across the country; others are new, sometimes controversial, and may require treatment in a specialized antenatal centre. This appendix also includes a discussion of antenatal diagnostic tests and procedures for ending an impaired pregnancy.

Genetic and Chromosomal Problems

The accidental rearrangement, realignment, or numeric changes in the twenty-three pairs of chromosomes in each cell, such as with Down's Syndrome, are called 'chromosomal' abnormalities. 'Genetic' anomalies can be traced to one or more of the one hundred thousand genes, or chemicals within the chromosomes that store information about bodily characteristics such as sex or eye colour and include such disorders as Tay-Sachs disease and haemophilia. Both chromosomal and genetic abnormalities can cause defects in a baby and pregnancy loss.

Probable Treatment
Chromosomal and genetic defects are not preventable. The adverse effects of certain genetic defects are treatable, but many are not. Once a genetic or chromosomal defect has been determined, the couple may want to consult a geneticist about the probability of the same problem recurring and about tests that can reveal its presence in a subsequent pregnancy.

Some chromosomal irregularities that lead to pregnancy loss can be discovered in the parents' bloodstreams or in fetal tissue. In either case, the chromosomal arrangement within the individual cells is photographed and examined in a procedure called karyotyping.

Hormonal Problems

Some hormonal problems can be determined by a blood test. Endometrial biopsy is the most effective method of determining the presence of the major hormonal imbalance, called luteal phase defect or LPD. If the uterine lining seems to be improperly developed for the day of the cycle on which it was gathered, the assumption is that a luteal phase defect is responsible. A single endometrial biopsy can misrepresent this condition, so two biopsies from two separate cycles are usually compared. A luteal phase defect is accompanied by low progesterone levels and occasionally by elevated levels of prolactin. These hormonal imbalances probably impede implantation of a fertilized egg.

Probable Treatment
Some of the drugs used to correct hormonal imbalances are considered controversial, and their use should be evaluated carefully for possible side effects. Clomiphene citrate, marketed under the brand name Clomid, is one of the major fertility drugs used in treating LPD because it increases progesterone levels. Progesterone injections or vaginal suppositories are also used, although the effectiveness of these treatments has not been clinically proven.

The primary treatment for prolactin imbalances is a drug called bromocriptine, which does not cure the causes of elevated prolactin but reduces levels for as long as it is taken, usually up to ovulation or through conception.

Uterine Problems

Uterine malformations can interfere with a growing pregnancy in a number of ways, some of which are more readily treatable than others. The major uterine disorders and their treatments are:

Abnormally Shaped Uteri

About one in every seven hundred women has some uterine abnormality that developed before she was born. Instead of the normal, pear-shaped uterus, these women may have a heart-shaped uterus, a uterus divided in half by tissue called a septum, or a T-shaped uterus. Any of these abnormalities might cause miscarriage by preventing the uterus from expanding properly to accommodate the pregnancy.

Probable Treatment
Only the divided uterus can be treated successfully with surgery to remove the separating tissue, although some experimental operations are being developed for other malformations. Many women with a septum can sustain healthy, full-term pregnancies, so doctors usually recommend surgery only after miscarriages attributed to the presence of the septum have occurred.

Fibroids

Between 10 and 20 percent of all women develop benign growths called myomas or fibroid tumours in the uterine muscle structure. Elevated hormone levels in a pregnant woman can cause some fibroids to grow excessively, changing the architecture of the uterus and interfering with implantation or growth of the pregnancy.

Probable Treatment
Most fibroids are harmless and can be detected during the regular gynaecological examination. There are two choices if the doctor decides the fibroids should be treated. One is drug therapy, to shrink the fibroids, which tend to return after treatment has been stopped. The other is surgical removal, which is usually performed by an incision through the abdomen and uterus.

Scarring and Adhesions

Excessive scarring and bandlike adhesions, also known as Asherman's Syndrome, can build up on the inside surface of the uterus, making it incapable of nourishing an implanted embryo.

Probable Treatment
With newly developed microsurgical techniques, removal of the scarring can be effective, allowing the uterus to regenerate its lining. However,

pregnancies occurring after this corrective surgery has been performed show an increased incidence of complications, including premature labour.

Immunological Problems

The three primary forms of immunological disorders that occur in pregnant women are:

Antiphospholipid Antibody Syndrome

This disorder, also known as the lupus anticoagulant, occurs when the mother's immune system turns against its own cells and tissues, including a developing placenta. The lupus anticoagulant can also cause blood clots to form within the placenta and may be responsible for as much as 10 percent of recurrent miscarriages. The disease can be determined by the amounts of antiphospholipid antibody in the mother's bloodstream.

Probable Treatment
One aspirin a day is the most common drug given, followed by aspirin in combination with prednisone, a steroid, or heparin, a blood thinner.

Lupus

Systemic lupus erythematosus, or SLE, is an autoimmune disorder in which the immune system begins to attack normal parts of the body. The cause is unknown. There are a variety of symptoms, including hair loss, specific rashes, light sensitivity, and inflammation, but no single test for this condition is conclusive. Pregnant women with lupus have a higher than average rate of both miscarriages and birth defects and often experience flare-ups during pregnancy or following birth. Lupus can be quite disabling and even lifethreatening.

Probable Treatment
With neither a cause nor a cure at hand, lupus is difficult to treat. Some of the symptoms can be controlled by rest, diet, and drugs, such as anti-inflammatory agents and steroids, both of which can have serious side effects. Some gynaecologists are not familiar with lupus, so a woman who wishes to become pregnant and either knows or suspects she has the disease should consult her specialist who will probably refer her to an obstetrician with experience of lupus pregnancy, usually in teaching hospitals.

Fetal Rejection

Problems can occur when the mother's body attacks the fetus as if it were a foreign object, such as a transplanted heart or kidney. In healthy pregnancies this immunological response is suppressed. However, if signals from the father's genetic material are too similar to the mother's, this suppression may not occur, and the pregnancy is attacked.

Probable Treatment
The treatment for fetal rejection is still controversial and is doubted by some respected doctors; however, it is being pursued by several hospitals in Britain, the USA and Europe. The goal is to trigger the protective immune response from the mother by giving her the appropriate signals, or antigens, during her pregnancy. These antigens are drawn from her husband's or another donor's blood and are injected before and during the pregnancy, 'vaccinating' her against possible rejection of her fetus. The programmes have not been in operation long enough to document possible long-term consequences on babies born following the procedure. See Appendix D for a list of hospitals in Britain that have information about immunotherapy treatment.

Premature Labour

Mothers who have experienced a loss from premature labour will probably be treated with strong medications, called tocolytics, after the twentieth week of a subsequent pregnancy, to curb uterine contractions. Current studies indicate that only the mothers experience the immediate side effects from tocolytics, but possible long-term effects on the off-spring are still unknown.

The drugs used to help stop premature labour are administered by one or more of several methods: orally, by injection into a muscle, by injection under the skin, and through an intravenous solution. The success of tocolytic drugs depends greatly on early diagnosis and treatment of premature labour. The most commonly used tocolytics include:

Ritodrine (Yutopar)
Helps inhibit the contractility of the uterine smooth muscles. It causes an elevated heart rate and other potentially serious side effects that should be monitored closely.

Salbutamol

An asthma medication that is very similar to ritodrine in chemical structure. It, too, increases the heart rate and can lead to bouts of nausea, nervousness, and other side effects.

Indomethacin

Primarily used as an anti-inflammatory agent in the treatment of rheumatoid arthritis. Since it also inhibits the hormone prostaglandin, it can slow labour. Use of this drug can cause side effects in the mother's gastrointestinal tract and eyes, as well as serious adverse effects in the fetus, including heart problems and a reduction in amniotic fluid. It is now rarely used.

Cervical Incompetence

Once a diagnosis of cervical incompetence has been established, the treatment is cervical cerclage. The most common procedure is the *Shirodkar* cerclage, in which a band of material is placed around the circumference of the cervix. It is accomplished through the vagina, but some techniques, for more serious cases, require an incision in the abdomen. Abdominal cerclages are usually performed between pregnancies and are considered permanent, so caesarean deliveries are necessary for subsequent pregnancies. In certain situations abdominal cerclages are performed after the pregnancy has been confirmed.

Maternal Illness as a Factor

Illnesses and medical complications that most women would normally endure without much worry can be sources of extreme danger to a baby, causing both birth defects and pregnancy loss. No medications for any disease or condition, even over-the-counter remedies, should be taken during pregnancy without consulting a doctor first. The following list is not a complete survey of all conditions and treatments that might be harmful to a pregnancy, but it demonstrates the vigilance pregnant women must maintain.

Diabetes

Diabetes is caused by the body's inability to produce enough insulin, resulting in high blood glucose levels, which in turn can cause a variety of metabolic problems. Diabetes in the mother used to be a frequent cause of birth defects, as well as causing excessive growth of the baby while in the womb. It can also lead to the production of too much amniotic fluid. Diabetic mothers have a higher risk of preeclampsia, miscarriage, stillbirth, and premature births. During pregnancy some women develop 'gestational diabetes,' which disappears after delivery.

Treatment

Pregnancy in diabetic patients requires a considerable amount of commitment. It is risky and involves constant monitoring, usually at a specialized medical centre. Treatment of a diabetic pregnancy may involve dietary modification, insulin injections, and home monitoring of blood glucose levels. Certain antenatal tests, such as that for alphafetoprotein and triple test will require special evaluation. As long as diabetics remain vigilant throughout pregnancy, the prognosis for delivering a healthy baby is almost as good as for other patients. Paternal diabetes seems to have no bearing on the father's offspring.

Hypertension

Hypertension, or high blood pressure, is one of the leading causes of midterm and late losses. It can also pose a danger to the mother.

This illness takes two forms during pregnancy. The first is when the mother had high blood pressure before the pregnancy. This condition can predispose her to the second type of hypertension, preeclampsia.

Preeclampsia can develop during the latter half of pregnancy in women who may or may not have had previous hypertension. Symptoms include high blood pressure, protein in the urine, and swelling due to fluid retention. The mother is at risk for convulsions and potentially fatal haemorrhaging.

Treatment

For pre-existing hypertension, the mother's need for bed rest and blood pressure medication is closely monitored during her pregnancy.

The only treatments for preeclampsia are bed rest and observation. If symptoms worsen, the baby must be delivered.

Measles, Mumps, Rubella, and Chickenpox

All four childhood viral diseases are generally rare in adults in developed countries because of the high incidence during childhood and vaccination, both of which lead to immunity. Of the four, rubella, also known as German measles, is the most dangerous if contracted by a pregnant woman. It can cause severe birth abnormalities, including mental retardation and deafness, as well as miscarriage and stillbirth. Chickenpox, also called varicella, has been occasionally implicated in premature labour and birth defects.

Treatment

A woman who wishes to become pregnant should be given a blood test to screen for these immunities before conception. If she is not immune, she should be vaccinated. The vaccines, which contain non-infectious live viruses, are generally not administered during pregnancy. A chickenpox vaccine is not currently available, and women who have not had the disease should avoid exposure during pregnancy.

PKU

Phenylketonuria, or PKU, is a genetic disorder that renders its victims incapable of metabolizing phenylalanine, an amino acid that is present in all protein foods, including meats and some vegetables. Unless PKU is treated, toxic levels of the amino acid accumulate in the blood, causing severe mental retardation. This outcome can be prevented with a low-phenylalanine diet, which has enabled many women with the disorder to reach childbearing age and contemplate pregnancy. Ordinarily the low-phenylalanine diet is not necessary for adults afflicted with PKU, but pregnancy is an exception. High phenylalanine levels are passed from mother to baby in amounts the fetus cannot handle effectively, causing birth defects and possibly miscarriages. Babies born of non-PKU mothers are routinely tested for this ailment in most hospitals so effective treatment can begin immediately.

Treatment

Women with PKU should resume a low-phenylalanine diet as soon as they begin to contemplate pregnancy and should maintain the diet throughout pregnancy. Aspartame, the low-calorie sweetener known by the brand name

NutraSweet, found in many diet foods and drinks, releases phenylalanine once it is ingested, so it should be avoided by all women with PKU.

Toxoplasmosis

Toxoplasmosis, which causes fever and flu-like symptoms, is produced by a parasite sometimes found in raw meat or the faeces of cats that have ingested infected rodents. Once infected, individuals become immune; however, over 60 percent of childbearing-age women have never contracted the disease. The highest risk from infection is from conception to the twenty-fourth week of pregnancy, when serious problems, including birth defects and some chance of miscarriage, can result. Immunity to toxoplasmosis can be detected by a simple blood test that is becoming more routine prior to conception.

Treatment

Once diagnosed, toxoplasmosis is treatable with antibiotics, some of which are safe to take during pregnancy and may reduce the likelihood of the infection passing to the baby. Detection during pregnancy involves potentially dangerous tests. Prevention in non-immune women is difficult but can be helped by not eating undercooked meat, by avoiding cat faeces, and by thorough hand-washing.

Urinary Tract Infections

Urinary tract infections are common complications during pregnancy. If left untreated, they can cause serious kidney ailments that have been implicated in premature labour, low birth weight, and newborn death. Accompanying high fevers might also be dangerous to a pregnancy. Sometimes symptoms, such as pain upon urination, or a need to urinate frequently, do not appear.

Treatment

Doctors should check a pregnant woman's urine for the presence of bacteria. If an infection is present, antibiotic treatment is necessary to prevent the bacteria from growing and developing into more serious kidney complications. Although some antibiotics are not recommended during pregnancy, others are considered quite safe, especially if weighted against the potential damage to the baby if an infection goes untreated.

Sexually Transmitted Diseases

Sexually transmitted diseases, or STDs, fall into two basic categories: those that cause pelvic inflammatory disease, or PID, and those that do not.

PID-Related Invaders

The most common and dangerous organisms are Gonorrhea, Chlamydia, and Mycoplasma, all of which have been implicated in premature rupture of the membranes and late miscarriage. All can be treated with antibiotics following accurate diagnosis, an often difficult task since infection is frequently symptomless. Because Mycoplasma in particular is difficult to culture and identify, some doctors treat couples who have experienced multiple early miscarriages with one of the broad-spectrum antibiotics known to kill this organism.

Non-PID Invaders

Three of the more common sexually transmitted diseases that do not cause PID are AIDS, syphilis, and herpes.

AIDS. Acquired immune deficiency syndrome, or AIDS, is a deadly virus that is spread through the exchange of blood or by semen. Women contract AIDS by either sharing a syringe or having sex with an infected partner. Before the AIDS virus was eliminated from blood supplies, it was also transmitted through transfusions and blood products. A woman who thinks she might have been exposed to the virus should have a blood test to determine if she has AIDS virus antibodies.

Syphilis. If syphilis is given the opportunity to go through all three of its phases, it ultimately attacks nearly every organ and tissue in the human body. In pregnant women, syphilis has been linked to premature labour, stillbirth, newborn death, and birth defects. Proper treatment with penicillin or other antibiotics can stop the advancement of and even cure syphilis, and a routine blood test can detect its presence.

Herpes simplex. Herpes is a common viral infection that can be transmitted through sexual contact. The body harbours the virus for an indefinite period, causing recurrent episodes of infection. Babies contract herpes as they pass through an infected birth canal, and a first-time infection in the mother after the twentieth week of pregnancy can lead to miscarriage or premature labour. An antiviral drug called acyclovir is used to treat herpes in adults, as well as newborns who contract herpes at birth.

Acyclovir has not been thoroughly tested for use during pregnancy, but considerable experience has been amassed, and it is probably safe.

Age as a Factor

Women are now waiting to start families until their careers are established, but there is an unfortunate consequence: The older the mother, the greater the risk of pregnancy loss from chromosomal problems or other causes.

Because a female is born with all the eggs she will ever release in her lifetime, she is likely to have some eggs that are poorly developed, that have been subjected to environmental hazards, or that have deteriorated over the years. If these eggs are fertilized, they do not have the internal structure to develop into a healthy fetus and will miscarry. Older mothers may be more prone to pregnancy loss because their hormonal system's ability to function properly might decrease with age. Diabetes and high blood pressure, two factors implicated in pregnancy loss, are also more common in older women.

Less research has been done on the effect of paternal age in pregnancy loss, but one study indicated an increased risk in fathers over fifty for defects other than Down's Syndrome.

Exercise as a Factor

For centuries, women adhered to the custom of 'confinement' during pregnancy, a kind of informal house arrest and enforced lack of physical activity. Being normally active during a healthy pregnancy is not dangerous to your developing baby. Check with your doctor, however, about the safety of vigorous exercise or new exercise regimens. If your pregnancy is a high-risk one, your doctor may recommend limiting your physical activity.

Antenatal Diagnostic Tests

The following tests may be used to diagnose problems in pregnancies:

Alpha Fetoprotein Analysis

Maternal serum alpha fetoprotein, or MSAFP, analysis is done with a blood sample of the mother between the fifteenth and twentieth weeks of the pregnancy. This test can detect neural tube defects in an unborn baby, which occur in one of every five hundred to one thousand pregnancies. The two most common defects are spina bifida, a condition that often results in mild to severe neurological impairment, and anencephaly, a fatal structural defect of the baby's skull and brain.

AFP is a protein in the serum, or body fluid, of the baby. Normally it is excreted in small amounts by the baby, is passed via the placenta to the mother, and can be measured in the mother's blood. When the neural tube around the spinal cord of the baby has failed to close properly, the open area 'weeps' AFP in much larger quantities than normal, and it is found at a higher level in the mother's blood.

However, a high maternal serum AFP reading alone cannot give a definitive diagnosis of neural tube defects. If a problem is suspected, the test is repeated. If MSAFP levels remain high, the woman is referred for a scan to determine if a neural tube defect is present. Amniocentesis may be suggested to check how high the levels of AFP are in the amniotic fluid.

Triple Test

Triple test is now undertaken in a number of hospitals instead of MSAFP testing and it is used to screen for Down's Syndrome as well as neural tube defects. A blood sample is taken from the mother between 16–20 weeks of pregnancy. The levels of two hormones, unconjugated oestriol and human chorionic gonadotrophin (HCG), are measured in addition to that of AFP. The test will pick up four out of five babies with spina bifida and almost all babies with anencephaly. In addition, the test will pick up two out of every three babies with Down's Syndrome. Results take approximately five working days (depending on the hospital) and are presented either as 'screen negative' or 'screen positive'. A screen negative means that there is less than a 1 in 250 risk of a Down's baby and that a neural tube defect is unlikely. A 'screen positive' result means that either there is an increased risk of a neural tube defect or that the risk of Down's Syndrome is greater than 1 in 250. The appropriate 'odds' are usually quoted in both cases. It is important to stress that this is a screening test, not a diagnostic test. A screen positive result does not therefore mean that a woman is carrying a handicapped baby – it simply means that further testing is advised. Similarly, a screen negative result does not guarantee a healthy baby – there is still a risk, even though it is a small one.

Amniocentesis

The most common procedure used for genetic testing is amniocentesis. This is the withdrawal of amniotic fluid, along with fetal cells, to examine the cells' genetic makeup. The procedure is done between the sixteenth and twentieth weeks of the pregnancy. The doctor visualizes the baby's position by ultrasound, then inserts a needle through the mother's abdomen into the amniotic sac and withdraws some fluid. It is important for the *entire procedure* to be done under ultrasound guidance, as babies can move and change positions quickly. A local anaesthetic is very occasionally used to numb the site where the needle will be inserted. The sensation felt as the needle enters may be of pressure or of slight pain.

Uterine cramping may occur during amniocentesis. In addition, uterine cramping and spotting often occur for a day or two after the procedure and obstetricians recommend that a woman rest as much as possible and avoid any overexertion for a couple of days after having an amniocentesis.

Fetal cells from the fluid must be cultured and examined before results are available, a process that takes between one and three weeks. About 1 percent of the time a culture does not grow and the test must be repeated, creating an additional delay.

There is controversy in the medical field about the chance of amniocentesis causing pregnancy loss; the precise reasons why it may cause losses are not really known. A loss probably occurs in about one in two hundred to one in four hundred procedures as a result of amniocentesis. The risk is likely to be on the lower end of the scale if amniocentesis is done at a tertiary referral centre that specializes in the procedure or by an obstetrician who performs amniocentesis frequently. In other words, the more experienced the practitioner who does the test, the better.

Chorionic Villus Sampling

Chorionic villus sampling (CVS) is a method of obtaining cells from the developing placenta in the first trimester of pregnancy. Since the placenta is derived from the fertilised egg, its cells show the genetic make-up of the developing baby.

There are two kinds of CVS procedures currently being undertaken, transabdominal and transcervical. The more usual one in Britain is the transabdominal procedure. The tissue is obtained by passing a needle through the abdominal wall under ultrasound guidance, just like amniocentesis, to obtain cells from the placenta.

A few centres in Britain, and almost all centres in many European countries, use the transcervical procedure. Tissue is obtained by means of a slim, sterile tube or catheter inserted through the woman's cervix. Slight suction is applied to the catheter to obtain the cells. In both cases, the procedure lasts about ten minutes. It may be slightly uncomfortable but is not painful. Transabdominal CVS has been shown to be slightly safer than the transcervical method, although as with all these procedures, it is operator skill that counts for most, whatever the procedure.

CVS is not as widely used as amniocentesis because of its slightly higher miscarriage rate. However, since most spontaneous losses occur in the first trimester of pregnancy, the true rate of loss caused by CVS is somewhat difficult to establish. The risk is generally quoted as 4 percent, although some studies quote only a 1 percent increase over the risk normally quoted for amniocentesis of 0.5–1 percent. In addition, there is a risk of about 1–2 percent of the results being ambiguous and of the woman having to be referred for amniocentesis as well.

Many prospective parents prefer CVS to amniocentesis as CVS can be performed early in the pregnancy, with results available within one to two weeks. If the couple is told of a problem, and decides to end the pregnancy, it will be a first trimester termination – usually emotionally less traumatic and medically far safer than a late termination.

Medical Procedures for Ending an Impaired Pregnancy

Dilatation and Curettage

In a D&C, the cervix is dilated and gently suctioned first to remove most of the products of conception. Then a long metal instrument with an open spoon-shaped tip is inserted into the uterus, and the sides are gently scraped of placenta or uterine lining. A D&C is usually performed up to twelve weeks of pregnancy.

Dilatation and Evacuation

At later gestation, a D&E may be done in some hospitals. Laminaria sticks, which dilate the cervix, are inserted into the vagina the night before the procedure. The next day the woman is usually given local anaesthesic. A suction pump, somewhat like a gentle vacuum, removes the uterine lining and the pregnancy. The woman can usually go home the same day the procedure is done and can expect a rapid physical recovery. However, the baby is not delivered intact, which some women find distressing.

Induction of Labour

Three different methods are most frequently used for inducing labour:

- Syntocinon, a hormone that starts uterine contractions, is administered to the woman intravenously.
- Prostaglandin suppositories or laminaria sticks are inserted vaginally.
- A needle is inserted through the woman's abdomen, amniotic fluid is withdrawn, and either a saline solution or a hormone that will start labour is injected into the amniotic sac, although this procedure is now less commonly used.

When labour is induced, the procedure may take from 24–36 hours. As with any labour, it is painful, but medication is available to ameliorate the pain. Women who go through this ordeal usually find the presence of their partner or another support person extremely helpful.

APPENDIX B

....

RITUALS

Planning a goodbye ritual for your baby may be one of the saddest tasks you will ever have to perform. But putting the time and effort into creating a tender, meaningful farewell can give you the chance to release and share your grief. A ritual can help begin the healing process and engender memories you will cherish for a lifetime.

Whether you write your own poems and prayers for your baby, ask a sensitive member of the clergy to create a ritual, or use some of the ceremonies suggested here, try to keep several issues in mind. Ask that your baby be mentioned by name. Using the baby's name and referring to the infant as 'he' or 'she,' 'our daughter' or 'our son,' can help you grasp your loss and move through your grief. If your loss was too early to know the baby's gender, try referring to the child as 'our infant' or 'our baby.' Mentioning the baby specifically and personally will also help friends and relatives who attend the service understand the magnitude of your loss.

In deciding what should be said at the service, consider sharing the dreams and hopes you had for your child, since you will not have a lifetime of memories to cherish. Allowing time for friends and family to speak or to read poems or selections they have chosen can add to the feeling of community during a service. If your ritual will be held in the hospital, consider inviting members of the medical staff who cared for you or your infant. There could also be time for people to hold hands during the service, or even hug one another. Many bereaved parents and their loved ones have found physical expressions of emotions and support during a memorial service both freeing and inspiring.

It can be important to acknowledge negative feelings toward God and your faith, as well as the comfort you may feel, during the service. Only by recognizing anger, guilt, and frustration can these emotions ever be overcome. Certain passages from Scripture, such as Psalm 51, express the sense that God understands sorrow and anger and accepts our feelings, no matter what they are.

You may want to incorporate symbols and gestures into your service that have particular meaning to you, for instance, the lighting of candles or release of helium ballons.

Whatever form your personal ritual takes, trust your own instincts and judgments. This was your pregnancy and your baby. It should be your goodbye as well.

Choosing a Place

If your baby is to be cremated or buried, a simple service may be held in the hospital chapel or a funeral home, with another brief prayer and Scripture reading at the grave or the site where the baby's ashes (if there are any) are to be scattered. Parents who are members of a congregation may want to have a more formal service in their regular house of worship; others prefer to gather in an informal setting, such as their own home or garden, for their baby's service.

If there is no burial, you may still wish to hold a service. If the baby was cremated and you choose not to scatter the ashes, you may also wish to hold a service. Some parents decide to scatter the ashes at a later time or reserve a portion of the ashes to bury with themselves eventually or to keep with them in case they move from their current home.

Including Grandparents

Including the baby's grandparents during a ritual can be a tender and effective way of acknowledging their particular grief, especially if they did not have the opportunity to see their grandchild. They could be asked to read a special prayer, Scripture, or poem. It is wise to be considerate of the feelings of relatives, especially grandparents, who may have specific expectations about a service because of their religious convictions. Recognizing the family's faith during the service is another way of expressing your desire to be consoled by your community.

Other Ways to Ritualize Your Grief

If you wish to acknowledge your baby's importance within a spiritual context but prefer to have the hospital or a religious society handle the burial, you may simply incorporate private prayers in a house of worship during a weekly service or on a special religious holiday. Jews might want to say Kaddish at any religious service, including Yiskor, the service that especially honours departed loved ones on major holidays such as Yom Kippur. Christians might choose All Saint's Day, an Easter service, or a candle-lighting ceremony at Christmas. You could ask a member of the clergy to remember your baby in his own private devotions or during his weekly pastoral prayer to the congregation.

Another way of giving expression to your grief is to create a memory book for your baby. Some of the organizations listed in the 'Resources' section of this appendix offer books specifically designed for this purpose. A simply designed baby book or a plain album you could title *Baby Memories* would be effective. Some families prefer small, delicate wicker baskets or ornamental boxes that can be filled with baby mementoes. Depending on how far advanced your pregnancy was before you experienced your loss, you might consider including:

- an early scan picture
- a copy of other antenatal test results, such as a photo of the baby's chromosomes from amniocentesis
- footprints
- a lock of hair
- birth certificate
- hospital ID bracelet
- letters of condolence
- list of baby presents
- a dried, pressed flower (this could also be framed) from the funeral
- photographs of the baby
- a copy of the memorial or funeral service and any poems or prayers that were read to the baby
- art work created by family and friends in honour of the baby, such as drawings made by an older sibling, or embroidery done by a loving grandmother.

Creating a Ritual

The rituals provided here are meant to be a point of departure for developing something personal for your own needs and faith traditions.

All of these prayers, Scripture readings, musical selections, and blessings can be adapted to early losses as well as late losses, to Jewish beliefs as well as to Christian concepts. If you do not have a member of the clergy present, a relative or friend could take the part of the 'leader' or 'friend.' Even parents who have grown away from their faith over the years, or who are in marriages of mixed religions, may find a ritualistic expression of their sorrow comforting and meaningful, especially if they help design it themselves.

The elements of the ritual may be arranged in any order that seems suitable, but here is a suggested format that would last about half an hour:

> *Musical selection* playing as people gather
> *Prayer* by a member of the clergy
> *Scripture reading* by a relative or friend
> *Song or hymn* sung together
> *Reading* of poem by a parent
> *Reading* by a relative or friend
> *Naming or blessing* of the baby by a member of the clergy
> *Scripture* reading by a relative or friend
> *Prayer* by a member of the clergy
>> or
> *Responsive reading* led by a member of the clergy
> *Musical reading* led by a member of the clergy
> *Musical selection* for silent prayer
> *Blessing* of the parents by a member of the clergy
> *Song or hymn* sung together
> *Benediction* by a member of the clergy

Bible Scripture

Some parents prefer the older, traditional Bible translations, while others feel more comfortable using more modern versions. Jews may wish to use *the Tanakh*, a modern translation of the Hebrew Bible.

Holy Scripture

(from the shared Jewish and Christian tradition, in alphabetical order)

Ecclesiastes 3:1–11   'To everything there is a season...'

Genesis 1:1–12   The Creation, 'In the beginning God...'

Isaiah 43:1–4   'I have called you by name and you are mine.   . .'

Isaiah 49:15–16   'I will never forget you.   . .'

Jeremiah 1:4–6   God knows babies in the womb and consecrates them.

Jeremiah 31:13–17   God will turn mourning into comfort; God hears Rachel weeping for her children.

Job 1:21   'Naked I came out of my mother's womb.   . . The Lord giveth and the Lord taketh away.   . .'

Job 3:6–16   The nature of stillbirth

Job 6:2–3   The weight of grief

Joshua 1:9   Be strong and of good courage, do not be dismayed: God is with you wherever you go.

Psalm 23   We can be comforted as we walk through the Valley of the Shadow of Death, as God walks with us.

Psalm 42   A cry of despair can be a cry of faith; when you thirst for God.

Psalm 46   God is our refuge and strength, a very present help in trouble.

Psalm 51:1, 6, 8, 17   God will not despise a broken and contrite heart.

Psalm 139:1–17   God knows your feelings and God knows your baby.

Psalm 147:3–13   God knows all the stars by name and blesses children in the womb.

Zechariah 12:10–11   Mourning for a child is overwhelming.

Holy Scripture

(from the Christian tradition, in order of appearance in the Bible)

Matthew 5:5   'Blessed are those who mourn, for they shall be comforted.'

Matthew 11:25–30   'Come unto me, all ye that labour and are heavy laden, and I will give you rest.   . .'

Mark 10:13–17   'Let the little children come unto me.'

John 11:35   Jesus wept [and so can we].

John 14:18   'I will not leave you comfortless. I will come to you.'

John 19:28   'I thirst' as a symbol of extreme need and suffering; read with Psalm 42 and Revelation 7:17.

I Corinthians 13:4–13   The 'love' chapter; 'Love endureth all things . . . When I was a child. . .'

II Corinthians 1:3–5   God comforts us so we can comfort others; one of the secrets to healing is that in helping others you help yourself.

Hebrews 5:7–8   Jesus understood tears and learned from his own suffering.

Revelation 7:17   God will guide us to water and will wipe away our tears.

With thanks to SISTER JANE MARIE LAMB

Music

Including music in your goodbye ritual can provide the tender mood you wish to set for the baby's service. Depending on where you hold your ritual, there may be a piano or organ available; if not, an accomplished singer or guitarist can lead the group in song. Singing together can evoke the sense of community and support you need. If you prefer to listen to musical selections, many of the popular songs, show tunes, and classical pieces listed here are readily available on tape.

Classical Selections

J. S. Bach, 'Jesu, Joy of Man's Desiring'

Ludwig van Beethoven, 'Für Elise'

Ludwig van Beethoven, *Piano Sonata*, Op. 13, the 'Pathetique,' 2nd Movement

Leonard Bernstein, *Candide*, Act I, 'It Must Be So'; Candide learns that 'there is a sweetness in every woe'

Leonard Bernstein, *West Side Story*, Act I, 'One Hand, One Heart'; Tony and Maria sing 'Even death won't part us now'

Johannes Brahms, 'Cradle Song' known as 'Brahms' Lullaby'

Frédéric Chopin, *Prélude*, Op. 28, No. 7

Gabriel Fauré, *Requiem*, especially the 'Kyrie'

Engelbert Humperdinck, *Hansel and Gretel*, Act II, 'Evening Prayer' ('When at night I go to sleep...'

Gustav Mahler, *Kindertotenlieder* (Songs for Deceased Children), especially No. 4, 'Often I think you have only gone out and will return...'

Felix Mendelssohn, 'On Wings of Song'

Wolfgang Mozart, *Requiem* – especially the 'Lacrimosa,' 'Hostias,'

'Agnus Dei,' and 'Lux Aeterna' sections

Giacomo Puccini, *Suor Angelica*, 'Senza mamma, o bimbo, tu sei morto!' Angelica says goodbye to her baby who died

Henry Purcell, *Dido and Aneas*, 'Dido's Lament' from Act III; Dido asks to be remembered after death

Maurice Ravel, *Pavane* ('On the death of an infant...')

Camille Saint-Saëns, *Carnival of the Animals*, especially 'The Swan' and 'Aquarium'

Franz Schubert, 'Ave Maria'

Franz Schubert, *Death and the Maiden*, either the song or String Quartet No. 14, 2nd Movement

Robert Schumann, *Scenes from Childhood*, especially 'From Foreign Lands and People,' 'Traumerei (Dreaming),' and 'Child Falling Asleep'

Richard Strauss, *Four Last Songs*, especially No. 3

Giuseppe Verdi, *Otello*, 'Ave Maria' from Act IV; Desdemona beseeches Mary to 'pray for those who bow their heads beneath outrage and misfortune'

Popular Music

'You'll Never Walk Alone' (from *Carousel*)

'Somewhere Out There' (from *An American Tale*)

'Let There Be Peace on Earth' (traditional)

'Blessed Are' (by Joan Baez)

'Turn, Turn, Turn' (from Ecclesiastes, adapted by Pete Seeger)

'Wings of a Dove' (by Bob Ferguson)

'Both Sides Now' (by Judy Collins)

'It's All Right to Cry' (by Carol Hall)

'You Have to Hurt' (by Carly Simon)

'In My Life' (by John Lennon and Paul McCartney)

Christian Hymns and Spirituals

'What a Friend We Have in Jesus'

'Still, Still with Thee'

'Amazing Grace'

'O Lord, Turn Not Thy Face from Them'

'The Day Thou Gavest, Lord, Is Ending'

'Blest Be the Tie That Binds'

'Jesus Loves Me'
'All Things Bright and Beautiful'
'Nearer, My God, to Thee'
'Be Thou My Vision'
'We Gather Together'
'Abide with Me'
'Jesus, Saviour, Pilot Me'
'Just As I am, Without One Plea'
'O God, Our Help in Ages Past'
'All My Trials'
'Rock of Ages, Cleft for Me'
'Now the Day Is Over'

Baptisms, Blessings, and Naming Rituals

Baptism is a sacrament of repentance and discipleship, a rite of passage for the living, and most members of the clergy feel it should not be applied to early losses or stillbirths. However, a blessing for a deceased baby can be worded so that the profound imagery of water inherent in baptism is maintained without the actual sacrament being given. This blessing can be combined with a naming ceremony.

The person officiating can describe the significance of water in this manner while blessing the baby:

Water, one of the most important elements of creation, is essential for human life in countless ways. In our grief it becomes the symbol of God's cleansing and forgiveness, the power of spiritual renewal, and the flow of life throughout the ages. With water we now bless this child:

O God of creation,
Your spirit moved over the waters of the universe
To create life in its first struggling forms.
You led your people through the waters of the seas to salvation.
Your power moves in the waters of the womb to hold and protect us.
Bless this baby [name] in your love. Amen.

We bathe this child in the love of God. We bathe this child in the tears of her parents. We know the power of water to permeate life and hold this child. The water of the womb sustained this child as the water of the universe and the power of God will hold her now. Amen.

Adapted and used with permission from SISTER MARY CLAIRE VAN ORSDAL, OSU

When combined with the naming of the baby, usually by asking the parents 'What name have you given your child?' this can be as powerful and comforting as baptism. The feeling of commitment to the baby can be especially strong if a naming certificate is completed and handed to the parents at the close of the service. Sister Jane Marie Lamb has established the custom of using a small seashell to hold water for blessing or baptizing a baby. When the ceremony is finished, the member of the clergy gives the seashell to the parents as a cherished keepsake.

Responsive Reading

Responsive reading is a powerful form of prayer that includes everyone who attends the service. A type of call and response or litany in which the 'leader' pleas for God's mercy followed by the group's unison recitation of a repeated reply, such as 'God, hear our prayer,' can evoke the sense of community and interaction so important in saying goodbye to your baby. The following responsive readings can be adapted to suit the needs of each bereaved family. Christians may say 'Jesus' for 'God.'

Responsive Reading After a Pregnancy Loss

Choose one of the following responses:

God, hear our prayer
Be with us, God
Thank you for being with us
We pray to God
You know our pain, God
God, grant us healing and strength
Hear us, Mother [or Father] God

Leader:
For the time of unending tears, pain, and struggle;
times of not being understood by family, friends,

times of longing and emptiness,
times of not being in control,
times of searching within and without.
We pray . . .
Response

Leader:

For all the memories of our baby;
for any brief moment of being with our baby,
for those who walked the journey of mourning with us,
for each time of remembering.
We pray . . .
Response

Leader:

For the times of letting go,
for the times of reaching out,
for each new day and each ray of hope,
for the gifts our baby left us:
in giving us new eyes with which to see,
new ears to help us hear others,
a new heart to love more deeply,
and for new values in our lives.
We pray . . .
Response

Adapted with permission from *Bittersweet . . . hellogoodbye* by

SISTER JANE MARIE LAMB

Prayers

Prayer Following Pregnancy Loss

May the Holy One who blessed our mothers
Sarah, Rebeccah, Rachel, and Linda,
bless and protect [name of mother].
May the wounds she has suffered,
both physical and emotional,
soon be healed.
May she find comfort in knowing

that You, O God, weep with her.
May the Source of Life,
the Creator of all flesh,
restore her body to its rhythms
and her soul to its songs of joy.
As she and [husband's name] stand before You
help them to move forward
to feel the pain,
acknowledge the loss
and move forward.
May all of us here be committed to living
always aware that we are created in Your image,
by caring, supporting, and loving one another
in times of pain as well as in times of joy.
As we have wept together,
so may we soon gather to rejoice together.
And let us all say
Amen.

by DIANE COHEN, used with permission

Prayer Following Pregnancy Loss

God, we know that [name of baby] is precious to you. Embrace her [him] in your loving arms. Tenderly comfort and strengthen those who mourn, especially the parents [names], the grandparents, [names of siblings], and all who mourn. We trust that you have heard our prayer.

Adapted with permission from *Bittersweet . . . hellogoodbye* by

SISTER JANE MARIE LAMB

Reading for a Miscarried Baby

Today we come together in sorrow over the death of _____ and _____'s baby. Their child, created in love and eagerly wished for, has died – never to be nestled securely in their arms in this lifetime. To these parents, the pain and the disappointment is great, and their loss will be carried heavily in their hearts in the weeks and months ahead. They will miss their child terribly and will be in need of love, compassion, time, and understanding from all of us.

Each life comes into this world with a mission. Sometimes the mission or purpose is clear; sometimes it is vague and shrouded in misunderstandings. In time, we will see what this baby's mission was on earth. Could it have been just to add a little flicker of love that otherwise may never have been lit? Was it to soften our hearts so that we may in turn comfort others? Could it have been to bring us closer to our God and each other?

This child's life was short, yet the death has left a huge void in all of our hearts and lives. Let us remember today and for always the tiny baby who will never see childhood or adulthood, but will remain our tiny baby forever.

SUSAN ERLING; reprinted with permission from *Planning a Precious Goodbye* by SHEROKEE ISLE, SUSAN ERLING, and MARY JO FLYNN and published by the Pregnancy and Infant Loss Center

Rituals Concerning Abortion

Prior to an abortion, the parents may want to set aside some private moments to say goodbye to their baby, to express their love and the deep sorrow they feel that the baby could not survive or would have lived with a diminished quality of life.

Act of Dedication After an Abortion

Leader:

God, Mother of us all, we ask Your blessing upon _____. Bless all who face the choice of abortion. Thank You for granting them the wisdom to make their choice and the courage to act upon it, all while embracing the knowledge of Your love. Grant unto all women the support and love we offer unto _____ this day and always. Bind us close in Your love and keep us faithful in our friendships. Hear our prayer, O God, our Mother and grant us mercy and forgiveness upon all our lives. Amen.

The mother may wish to read the following prayer:

The choice has been made.
One of the hardest of my life.
Bless me as I go forth.

Help me to face the guilt I feel
so that I may not run away from the truth.
Empower me to own the fear in my heart
that I may have compassion
for others who share my pain.
Bless all who support me
with the strength of their love;
In the name of God (Jesus Christ).
Amen.

The mother and father may wish to make an 'act of dedication,' individually or jointly in the name of their child, and ask for friends' support to keep their vow. The promise should be personal, specific, and attainable, such as, 'In the name of our child, we promise to give £____ every month for the coming year to support a homeless child,' or 'In the name of our child, we promise we will plant a garden on the street where all who pass by may see the abundance of God's grace.'

Prayer (as water is poured from a pitcher into a bowl placed in front of the woman):

Leader:

We pour this water as a symbol of the tears of mourning, the forgiveness of guilt, and the beginning of a new life for you. We beseech God to uphold you and to fill you with grace, that you may know the healing power of God's divine love. We give you our love, promising to stand by you now and through the days to come. Amen.

(At the end, friends greet one another with hugs, the sign of friendship and peace.)

Adapted from *Prayers of Our Hearts*, Copyright © 1991 by VIENNA COBB ANDERSON. Reprinted with the permission of The Crossroad Publishing Company, New York.

APPENDIX C
· · · · · · · · · · · · · · · ·

PREGNANCY LOSS AND THE ENVIRONMENT

As humankind learns to respond more effectively to the emotional needs of bereaved parents, it must also understand the larger issues that impact on pregnancy loss. Airborne pollutants, grinding poverty that denies pregnant women proper antenatal care, and certain exposures in the workplace and at home may all affect pregnancy outcome.

Until recently, doctors believed that a baby in the womb was completely protected by the mother's body. They incorrectly assumed that the placenta not only nourished the baby, but protected him as well, by filtering out harmful substances before they could reach the developing baby. As a result of this misconception, pregnant women were exposed to potentially toxic substances, including medications, in the belief that there would be no effect on their unborn babies.

History and research eventually demonstrated that unborn babies can be affected by environmental toxins or by medication given to the mother. Well-known examples include birth defects and pregnancy loss resulting from maternal exposure to the hormone diethylstilboestrol (DES), the anti-nausea drug thalidomide, and the chemical plant accident in Bhopal, India.

To protect our future children, it is necessary to think beyond just what the mother eats for nine months, or which diseases she might contract during pregnancy. We must consider the quality of the air she breathes and what pollutants the baby's father might have been exposed to at work.

It is incumbent upon us to stop or at least forestall increased damage to our environment and, ultimately, ourselves. We can become conscious of potential hazards and remove ourselves from their proximity as well as becoming vocal opponents of policies that allow incidents of reckless and hazardous exposure to occur. We can support politicians who enforce proper regulations of harmful substances, not just in our own backyard but worldwide as well. We must become advocates for a better-educated, more aware populace who can produce a cleaner, safer, more ethically managed planet and give all unborn babies a better chance at life.

The Mechanism of Exposure

Harmful substances can enter the body by being inhaled, ingested, or absorbed through the skin or mucous membranes; some radiations can penetrate the human body. Once in the body, these agents have an impact on the mother, father, or developing baby in one of several ways: (1) by damaging the structure of sperm, ova, or embryonic cells so they do not grow properly; (2) by altering the number or pairing of chromosomes within a cell; (3) by affecting the genetic material within the chromosomes; or (4) by compromising some bodily function in the baby or the mother.

Because human reproduction is such a complex, delicate, and interactive process, it is vulnerable to a number of harmful exposures in both parents even before they conceive a child. Researchers once believed that female ova were the primary casualties because they exist in an unborn baby girl's reproductive tract and must withstand a lifetime of potentially harmful exposures. It was also thought that only the heartiest sperm managed to reach and fertilize an egg, so any anomalies in the baby must have come from a defect in the ovum.

Although eggs can be affected by harmful exposures, it is now known that a genetically defective sperm can reach and penetrate a healthy egg. Because sperm divide rapidly before fertilization, they may be subject to additional genetic alterations as they grow, especially if the father has been exposed to environmental toxins.

As the unborn baby grows in the womb, it can be further imperiled by harmful materials, some of which are more hazardous than others, depending on the developmental stage of the baby at the time of exposure. Some exposures may occur after birth through the mother's breast milk; others, like DES, may not become evident until the child reaches sexual maturity. Risk assessment of potentially harmful exposures covers a much longer time frame than was previously recognized.

Once a hazardous agent does its damage, its impact on pregnancy is twofold: The baby may stop growing properly, triggering a miscarriage, or the unborn baby can develop a disorder that could lead to abnormalities, stillbirth, or neonatal death.

Substances

In 1961, after thalidomide was pulled from the market and the medical profession gained a clearer understanding of the role the placenta plays in transmitting substances to the developing baby, people began to wonder what other harmful elements might be passed through this extraordinary organ. Researchers discovered that most harmful substances, be they natural microorganisms or synthetic chemicals, pass through the placenta to the baby. They also noted that some substances harm the baby indirectly by impeding the placenta's functions. For a discussion of the impact of maternal illness and medications on pregnancy, see Appendix A.

Radiation

The emission of natural 'background' radiation from the sun and from radioactive minerals in the soil has been ongoing for millennia, but radiation remains one of the most misunderstood of all the potentially harmful agents. Radiation is the transportation of energy from one place to the other, and it takes two basic forms: pure energy waves such as light, radio waves, or radar; and energy made up of subatomic particles such as electrons. Seemingly harmless in its silence and unseen impact, radiation nevertheless can affect the atoms that make up the cells in human bodies, including those of unborn babies.

Our bodies are criss-crossed hundreds of times a day by radiation from both natural and manufactured sources. If a direct 'hit' is made in some necessary strand of DNA in an unborn baby's cell, which is not likely to happen from background radiation, it could lead to non-viability or a genetic problem, either of which could result in pregnancy loss.

All forms of radiation are further distinguished by their energy levels and fall into two groups: ionizing or particle radiation, in which the rays can break atoms into pieces, and non-ionizing radiation, which cannot. It is clear that ionizing radiation such as X-rays and gamma rays are harmful at high enough doses. The controversy is still blazing over the effects of non-ionizing radiation, the kind that is produced by most electrical appliances; these potential risks are discussed in greater detail below.

Depending on the elevation of our homes and the geographical distribution of radioactive minerals, we are all subjected to natural levels of background radiation. People who live in Cornwall, with its rocky outcrops of granite are at the high end of this spectrum. However, they do not have noticeably increased cancer rates or birth defects compared to people living elsewhere in the UK, where radiation levels are at the lower end of the scale. Clearly, levels of background radiation are not the only factors, and we must look further, to air- and waterborne pollutants, for health hazards as well.

Environmental Exposure and Your Next Pregnancy

Couples who are planning a pregnancy after a loss tend to be extremely cautious about any substance or activity that might be harmful. This is not unfounded, and parents are urged to be educated consumers. But keeping track of the controversies swirling around various exposures would be more than a full-time job and could cause unintentional worry about the new pregnancy as well as unnecessary guilt over a previous loss.

If you work with chemicals or radiation and have chronic exposure, your union and the organizations listed in the 'Resources' section of this appendix would be good sources of information and help. If, however, you are concerned about non-occupational exposure, you may want to keep a couple of issues in mind as you read reports in newspapers and magazines about potentially toxic exposures.

Cause and effect cannot be determined just from case reports or 'clusters' of incidences. Controlled scientific studies are always necessary. Although clusters of incidences may alert scientists to a serious problem, such as they did with thalidomide, they also tend to raise alarm and fear. They are never the final word, especially in situations that are as frequent and random as pregnancy loss. In reading reports about animal studies, you should also understand that large doses of any substance given to pregnant animals in laboratory tests do not necessarily correspond to most human exposures.

Risks vary, depending on how much exposure occurred, how long it continued, and when in the reproductive process it transpired. A continuously low level of exposure may or may not be just as damaging as a single catastrophic accident. Unfortunately, the risks of exposure cannot be identified until the harm has occurred, so conclusions are drawn painfully after the fact. And for many substances, tests are contradictory, inconclusive, or nonexistent.

The result is that everyone, especially pregnant women, should exercise reasonable prudence in avoiding certain exposures, even those that may be controversial. If you are pregnant, or want to be pregnant, and you believe you may be exposed to sources of hazardous materials at work or at home, you will need to weigh the potential risks against any inconvenience changing your situation might cause.

There are thousands of agents that can compromise the health of parents and their unborn children. Researchers do not agree on what degree of exposure constitutes a risk, so discussion of substances and agents may appear differently here than in other materials you may read.

Exposures With Known Risks

Many substances are regulated because they have a known detrimental effect on health, but none is governed solely on the basis of reproductive hazards. Only a few are restricted in the workplace, partially because of their known reproductive effects including ionizing radiation and lead. Products available for home use may have warnings on the labels, but it is up to the consumer to read them and take precautions – or risks. The following are exposures known to have a deleterious effect on pregnancy outcome based on conclusive documentation and current knowledge:

Alcohol definitely has an effect on pregnancy, but it varies with how frequently and how much is ingested, and at what point in the pregnancy it is consumed. No clear, safe level of alcohol consumption has been established for pregnant women. Women who drink heavily while pregnant run an increased risk of having miscarriages or giving birth to babies with fetal alcohol syndrome, which includes birth defects such as mental retardation and growth abnormalities. The safest course is to abstain from alcohol throughout pregnancy. If you are currently pregnant and drinking, abstaining at the earliest possible time can reduce the impact on the baby. If you are having trouble giving up alcohol, seek help from Alcoholics Anonymous or an alcoholism referral organization listed in your telephone directory.

Chemotherapy treatments while pregnant are risky, and the impact on the pregnancy depends on the dosages and combinations of drugs used. Since chemotherapy is designed to interfere with the rapid division of cells, there is a strong theoretical concern about using it during pregnancy. The impact on pregnant doctors and nurses who work with these drugs has not been thoroughly examined, but a recent study indicated that pregnant health-care professionals who handled these drugs in the first trimester had a statistically significant increase in miscarriages. Patients can have healthy pregnancies following certain chemotherapy treatments.

Lead is a toxic metal that accumulates in the body primarily through exposure to vehicle emissions and contact with old paint and plumbing. Its adverse effect on pregnancy is not known at low levels, but is confirmed at high levels of occupational exposure.

Smoking tobacco has long been implicated in the incidence of heart disease, lung disease, and cancer, but recent studies have also shown a correlation between smoking and an increase in miscarriage rates, stillbirth, placental separation, newborn death, and birth defects. Men who smoke tend to have lower sperm counts and a higher incidence of damaged sperm, which could lead to additional reproductive problems and loss. More research is needed to assess the relationship between nonsmokers who inhale other people's smoke and the health of unborn children, but the risks to the mother are so clear that a pregnant woman should not smoke or be around smokers. Stopping smoking at any point in the pregnancy reduces the impact on the baby. If you are having trouble quitting, contact the Quitline, a national telephone helpline for smokers who need help or advice in stopping, on 071–487–3000.

X-rays, as a type of ionizing radiation, should be used with caution during pregnancy. However, in a case of medical necessity where X-rays are the best diagnostic tool, a pregnant woman should feel safe having the examination as long as proper precautions are taken by a knowledgeable physician. Diagnostic X-ray exposures are generally very low. A woman who did not realize she was pregnant when she had a diagnostic X-ray should not seek an abortion without first getting an opinion from a specialist as it is extremely unlikely that diagnostic X-rays would harm the developing baby.

The standard 'dose' of X-rays involved in a chest X-ray is 20 msv – the same as you would expect to receive if you spent a day in Cornwall.

Exposures Suspected of Risks

Some substances have been subjected to studies, but the results have been flawed, contradictory, or inconclusive. Genuine concerns remain, and these agents deserve further scrutiny:

Caffeine is a stimulant that is a major ingredient in a number of foods, beverages, and over-the-counter medicines. Some studies have linked caffeine consumption to a greater risk of miscarriage, stillbirth, and premature birth, but the strong association between caffeine and cigarette smoking, which has definitely been proved harmful, may have skewed the results.

Cancer radiation therapy can be administered during pregnancy, but the amounts or radiation and the location of the cancer are critical in determining the danger to a developing baby. A woman in this situation, or one who wishes to conceive after treatment, should seek out the opinions of experts in both radiation oncology and fetal medicine, because effects on the baby could range from no damage to mild deformities, severe abnormalities, or fetal death.

Cocaine is a stimulant that can produce an intense euphoria or 'high.' It constricts the blood vessels, increases the heart rate, and causes a rise in blood pressure, all of which may affect the incidence of premature delivery, placental abruption, and the baby itself. The outcomes of some recent studies may be clouded by such factors as the incidence of poor nutrition and other drug use among cocaine users.

Glycol-ethers are a group of chemicals that are widely used in a number of products such as varnishes, spray lacquers, and metal-cleaning formulas, and in industry. Recent animal tests indicate glycol-ethers may have a potent effect on both male and female reproduction, but no extensive studies have been done in humans.

Mercury is a chemical that is accumulated in the body from environmental exposures and has been implicated in birth defects but not necessarily pregnancy loss. Mercury enters the water supply primarily through industrial wastes as inorganic mercury, is absorbed by fish, and is transformed into an extremely toxic, organic form of mercury, which is consumed with the fish. Accidental exposure to inorganic mercury by breaking a thermometer is not serious. There are no reliable studies on the risks of occupational exposure to inorganic mercury, used as a common amalgam in dentistry.

Power plants vary in hazards according to the source of power. Coal-burning plants are the most dangerous, since they output many harmful emissions into the air, including some radioactive material. Nuclear power plants are very highly regulated, and the radioactive emissions are considerably lower than those from coal plants. The danger from nuclear power plants comes from catastrophic accidents, such as the one in Chernobyl, and from the storage of radioactive waste products, a problem that has not yet been satisfactorily solved. Even alternative energy technologies are not without risk. Geothermal plants currently being developed and studied were once touted as a safe wave of the future, but by tapping into deep underground bubbling hot springs these facilities also release radon, a radioactive gas.

Exposures Whose Risks Are Unknown

Some exposures have been questioned because 'cluster' incidences of miscarriage have been noticed among certain groups of people. In other situations exposure to a hazardous agent is known, but increased risk of pregnancy loss has not been demonstrated. In either case, further scientific study is mandatory.

Electrical appliances produce non-ionizing electromagnetic radiation. Most of the sources of the radiation are either well sealed inside the appliances, as in microwave ovens, or are at the back, away from human proximity, as in television sets. If the intensity of radiation is high enough to produce a thermal effect on the human body, there is no question that it is harmful; there is some controversy over whether low levels cause damage. Electric blankets and heating pads are used in close proximity to humans for long, uninterrupted periods of time and may have more potential for harm. Although there is no current scientific evidence to support harm, pregnant women may want to exercise prudence until more is known about this type of exposure. For example, consider using an electric blanket to warm up a bed, but leaving it turned off while you are sleeping.

Extended air travel at high altitudes exposes people to additional radiation levels. Although the long-term effects have not been documented, people who travel extensively, including pilots and flight attendants, should be well informed of the risks of their exposure. Since the levels are similar to other radiation-related jobs, such as work at nuclear power plants, pregnant women and other employees should have as much knowledge as possible to make an informed decision about continuing to work under these conditions. Occasional air travel for business and pleasure while pregnant is probably safe.

Hair and nail care products, especially perms, dyes, nail polishes, and removers, contain chemicals commonly used by many people, but none of these products has been thoroughly evaluated for its effect on pregnancy. Women and men who work with these products and are contemplating pregnancy might want to wear rubber gloves and insist on well-ventilated working conditions.

Radio towers and high-tension wires emit non-ionizing radiation, but the hazards are not clear, and studies are still being conducted.

Radon is a light radioactive gas that permeates up through the soil from deposits of radium in the rocks below. It is a major source of background radiation exposure in certain parts of the UK, but its effect on pregnancy outcome is not known.

Video display terminals or computer monitors have been the subject of considerable controversy, but seven of eight recent studies showed no harmful effects on pregnancy. Like other appliances, computer monitors produce non-ionizing radiation; the magnetic coils that emit the radiation are usually in the rear of the terminal. Monitors vary in their emissions, depending on the manufacturer. A well-constructed monitor may emit less radiation from the back near the coils than a poorly made monitor emits from the front. Some manufacturers are now making emission information public. If you cannot find out the emissions level of your monitor, try to limit the number of hours you spend in front of the machine, and sit more than a foot and a half away, since the impact of radiation decreases greatly with distance. If you are still concerned, turn off the monitor completely (not just the screen) when not in use, and avoid sitting next to the back of another monitor. Manufacturers are aware of this problem and are making changes in their product designs to meet the emission guidelines used in Sweden, which are considered to be the more stringent.

Poverty and Pregnancy Loss

There has always been a strong correlation between unfavourable pregnancy outcome and the socioeconomic level of the mother. Analysts attributed part of this to the inadequacy of medical care available to impoverished pregnant women. Many studies have suggested that when better antenatal education is available, the incidence of low birth weight babies and perinatal death decreases.

It is hard to separate cause from effect in this complex issue. A pregnant woman who does not have access to good antenatal care may therefore not realize the impact smoking and alcohol, poor nutrition, or hazardous materials might have on her unborn child.

This prospect raises uncomfortable issues for our society as we try to grapple with a more equitable way of managing our planet. What we do now will have a far-reaching impact not only on the issue of pregnancy loss but also on our society as a whole.

RESOURCES

Books

When a baby dies, Nancy Kohner and Alix Henley, Pandora Press.
  Offers insight and information for parents whose babies have died.
Family, Susan Hill, Penguin. Discusses the birth, and subsequent death of
  Susan Hill's premature baby.
Miscarriage, women's experiences and needs, Christine Moulder, Pandora
  Press.
Miscarriage, stillbirth and neonatal death; guidelines for professionals, SANDS*.
A guide to effective care in pregnancy and childbirth, M Enkin, M Keirse and I
  Chalmers, Oxford University Press (paperback edition).
Helping children cope with grief, Rosemary Wells, Sheldon Press.
Thumpy's Story, Nancy Dodge, Prairie Press*.

Leaflets

After the death or stillbirth of your baby: what has to be done.
Saying goodbye to your baby. A guide for parents whose baby dies around
  the time of birth.
For Family and Friends. How you can help
The next pregnancy – guidance for parents
SAFTA – Support after Termination for Abnormality, Handbook.

*(available through SANDS)

Support for Parents

The Stillbirth and Neonatal Death Society (SANDS)

8 Portland Place, London W1N 4DE (071 436 5881).
For parents whose babies are born dead or die soon after birth

The Miscarriage Association

c/o Clayton Hospital, Northgate, Wakefield, W Yorks (0924 200799).
Information, advice and support for women who have had, or who are
having, a miscarriage. Local support groups

SAFTA (Support after Termination for Abnormality)

29 Soho Square, London W1V 6JB (071 439 6124).
Charity offering support for parents who have had, or are about to have, a
termination following a diagnosis of abnormality

Twin and Multiple Births Association (TAMBA)

PO Box 30, Little Sutton, S Wirral L66 1TH (051 348 0020).
For parents who have lost one or both twins or babies from a multiple birth.
TAMBA bereavement counselling details available through SANDS

Blisslink (also incorporates NIPPERS bereavement group)

17–21 Emerald St, London WC1N 3QL (071 831 9393).
For parents of babies in intensive and special care

The Foundation for the Study of Infant Deaths (FSID)

35 Belgrave Square, London SW1X 8PS (071 235 0965).
Support and information for parents bereaved by a sudden infant death
(Scottish equivalent, Scottish Cot Death Trust (041 357 3946)

National Childbirth Trust

Alexandra House, Oldham Terrace, Acton, London W3 6NH (081 992 8637).
Has local branches which can put parents in touch with someone who has
been through a similar experience

Other Helpful Addresses

Child (Infertility)

PO Box 154, Hounslow TW5 0EZ (081 893 7110).
Support organization for people coping with problems related to infertility, including loss after infertility

Issue

St George's Rectory, Tower Street, Birmingham B19 3UY (021 359 4887).
A support and information organization with similar aims to CHILD

Maternity Alliance (Benefits)

15 Britannia Street, London WC1X 9JP (071 837 1265).
Information on all aspects of maternity services. Particularly good on rights at work and benefits

Contact a Family

16 Strutton Ground, London SW1P 2HP (071 222 2695).
Comprehensive organization which maintains a directory of specific conditions and rare syndromes, together with information about each and how to contact other parents who have been through the same experience

Genetic Interest Group

Institute of Molecular Biology, John Radcliffe Hospital, Oxford OX3 9DU (0865 744002).
If your baby has died because of genetic disease, GIG will refer you to the appropriate organizations for counselling or further information

WellBeing (formerly Birthright)

27 Sussex Place, Regent's Park, London NW1 (071 262 5337).
Undertakes medical research into wide range of specific problems during pregnancy and birth. Can tell you whether research is being undertaken on the problem that affected your baby

Specific Conditions

APEC (Association for Pre-Eclampsia)

61 Greenways, Abbots Langley, Herts, WD5 0EV.
Has 24-hour helpline (0923 266778).

Association for Spina Bifida and Hydrocephalus (ASBAH)

42 Park Road, Peterborough, PE1 2UQ (07533 555988).
Also covers anencephaly

Cervical Stitch Network

Fairfield, Wolverton Road, Norton Lindsey, Warwickshire
For women having cervical cerclage in pregnancy

Heartline Association

12 Cremer Place, The Chestnuts, Wildish Rad, Faversham, Kent (0795 539864).
For parents of children born with heart disease. Has a bereavement group

Meningitis Research

Old Gloucester Road, Alverston, Bristol BS12 2LQ (0454 413344).
Offers counselling for parents whose babies die of meningitis

Counselling and Psychotherapy

British Association For Counselling

37a Sheep Street, Rugby, Warks CV2 3BX (0788 78328).
Information on where to get counselling locally

Compassionate Friends

6 Denmark Street, Bristol BS1 5DQ (0272 292778).
Support for parents of children who have died

CRUSE

Cruse House, 126 Sheen Road, Richmond, Surrey TW9 1UR (081 940 4818).
Support for the bereaved

London Bereavement Projects Co-ordinating Group

356 Holloway Road, London N7 6PN (071 700 8134).
Can refer people to local bereavement services

RELATE (Marriage Guidance)

Herbert Gray College, Little Church St, Rugby, Warks CV21 3AP (0788 573241).
Confidential counselling on relationship problems

Westminster Pastoral Foundation

23 Kensington Square, London W8 5HN (071 937 6956).
Offers individual and family counselling and can give information about availability of similar services elsewhere in the UK

GLOSSARY

Abortion, elective, therapeutic or voluntary: Deliberate ending of a pregnancy by medical intervention.

Abortion, spontaneous: See miscarriage.

Abruption, placental: Separation of the placenta from the uterine wall.

Adhesions: The scar tissue that binds together two surfaces that are usually apart.

AIDS (acquired immune deficiency syndrome): A fatal disease that affects the immune system and that can be transmitted through the exchange of blood or semen.

Alphafetoprotein: A protein produced by the fetus that can be measured prenatally to identify possible neural tube disorders.

Amniocentesis: The removal of a sample of amniotic fluid by means of a needle inserted through the mother's abdominal wall; used for genetic and biochemical analysis of the fetus.

Amniotic fluid: The liquid surrounding and protecting the baby within the amniotic sac during pregnancy.

Amniotic sac: The membrane within the uterus that contains the baby and the amniotic fluid during pregnancy.

Anencephaly: A fatal congenital condition in which most of the brain and skull are absent.

Anaesthesia: A gas or drug that causes partial or complete loss of sensation either in one part of the body (local) or with loss of consciousness (general).

Anniversary reaction: The resurgence of grief feelings and symptoms around a significant date following a loss. For a pregnancy loss this might be a due date or a delivery date.

Anomaly: A physical malformation or abnormality.

Antenatal: The period before birth and after conception

Antenatal diagnosis: The testing of a baby prior to birth.

Antibiotics: Medication that can eradicate or stop the growth of bacteria that attack humans.

Antibody: A substance produced in the body that attacks bacteria and viruses.

Artificial insemination: The injection of semen by syringe into the vagina, cervix, or uterus to fertilize an egg.

Asherman's syndrome: Uterine adhesions produced by infection or overly vigorous curettage of the uterus.

Autoimmune disease: The process in which the body's defense system acts against its own tissues, causing damage.

Bacteria: One-celled microorganisms. Some bacteria live in harmony with the human body, while others cause disease.

Bereavement (grief, mourning): The emotional state that accompanies a significant loss.

Bereavement, chronic or inhibited: The emotional state in which feelings of loss are not released and are pushed from consciousness, resulting in physical and psychological symptoms.

Beta subunit of HCG: See HCG.

Biopsy: The surgical removal of a small amount of tissue for microscopic analysis and diagnosis.

Birth control: The act of preventing conception through various methods.

Blighted ovum: See miscarriage.

Bonding: The emotional attachment of parents to their child, which can begin from confirmation of the pregnancy.

Calcification, placental: A condition in which excessive calcium in the placenta interferes with its functions.

Catheter: A slim tube used for removing or injecting fluids.

Cerclage: A surgical method for closing an incompetent cervix during pregnancy to prevent premature delivery. Also known as a 'stitch'.

Cervical incompetence: The condition in which a weakened cervix opens prematurely during pregnancy, sometimes resulting in pregnancy loss.

Cervix: The neck of the uterus leading to the vagina that opens during labour.

Caesarean section: The surgical removal of an unborn baby by means of an incision through the abdominal wall and the uterus.

Choriocarcinoma: A rare and highly treatable form of cancer that develops from placental tissue in about 15 percent of molar pregnancies.

Chorionic villus sampling: An antenatal test in which a soft, thin tube is inserted through the cervix, or a needle through the abdomen, to the chorionic villi, the embryonic tissue that forms the placenta, to withdraw a tissue sample for chromosomal and genetic analysis.

Chromosomal abnormality: A birth defect resulting from the accidental rearrangement of the chromosomes, as in Down's Syndrome.

Chromosomes: Structures found in human cells that contain genes, the material responsible for the transmission of hereditary information.

Climax: *See* orgasm.

Clomid: The brand name for clomiphene citrate, a synthetic hormone that stimulates the pituitary gland and ovulation.

Clomiphene challenge test: An analysis of the woman's response to doses of Clomid, which may be an indicator of her closeness to the onset of menopause and her ability to sustain a pregnancy.

Conception (becoming pregnant): The fertilization or union of egg and sperm to create a new life.

Cone biopsy: The surgical removal of a cone-shaped wedge of tissue from the cervix for microscopic analysis.

Congenital defect: A condition or abnormality that is present at birth, that may or may not be hereditary.

Contraception: *See* birth control.

Crisis pregnancy: A pregnancy that requires medical intervention including surgery, bed rest, induction of labour, or other treatments.

Culdocentesis: The insertion of a needle through the vaginal wall into the abdominal cavity behind the uterus to see if blood is present, indicating internal bleeding.

D&C (dilatation and curettage): Expansion of the cervix and suctioning to remove most of the products of conception, followed by gentle scraping of the uterine lining using a surgical instrument (curette) with an open, spoon-shaped tip, usually performed between conception and twelve weeks.

D&E (dilatation and evacuation): A procedure performed usually between the fourteenth and twentieth weeks of pregnancy in which the cervix is opened and the uterine contents removed by a suction device or by curettage.

DES (diethylstilbestrol): A synthetic form of oestrogen used from 1945 until the early 1970s principally in the USA and previously believed to prevent potential miscarriages. DES did little to forestall miscarriages and caused medical problems in children of mothers who took this hormone while pregnant.

DNA (deoxyribonucleic acid): A chemical compound within the gene that contains the genetic code.

Down's Syndrome: A common chromosomal birth abnormality with characteristic facial and other physical traits and differing levels of mental retardation.

Ectopic pregnancy: The implantation of a fertilized egg outside the uterus.

Efface, effacement: The thinning of the cervix during labour.

Embryo: The term used to describe a pregnancy from the fourth to the ninth week after conception.

Embryonic sac: The membrane within the uterus that contains the embryo.

Endocrine: The system of glands that secrete hormones.

Endometrial biopsy: The removal of a small sample of uterine lining, or endometrium, through the cervix, done for laboratory analysis between the twenty-first and twenty-fifth days of the menstrual cycle. Helps determine evidence of ovulation.

Endometriosis: A condition in which pieces of the endometrium, or uterine lining, are located outside the uterus.

Endometrium: The lining of the inner surface of the uterus.

Episiotomy: A surgical incision made during delivery that enlarges the external vaginal opening.

Fallopian tube: The thin, hollow conduit that carries the ovum, or egg, from the ovary to the uterus; named after the Italian anatomist Fallopius.

Fertilization: The penetration of the sperm into the ovum, or egg, to create a new life.

Fetal heart monitor: A small device that can be strapped to a pregnant woman's abdomen to evaluate the baby's heart rate.

Fetus: The term applied to a developing baby from nine weeks until birth.

Fibroid tumours (myomas): Non-malignant growths within the wall of the uterus that may expand during pregnancy.

Gene: The biological unit of a chromosome that carries inherited traits.

Genetic abnormality: A disorder resulting from an anomaly in the gene structure that is hereditary or that can occur as a spontaneous mutation.

Genetic counselling: The advice offered by experts in genetics on the detection, consequences, and risk of recurrence of chromosomal and genetic disorders.

Gestation: The period of fetal development in the womb from implantation to birth.

Grief: See bereavement.

Gynaecologist: A physician who specializes in the care of the female reproductive tract. The field is called gynaecology.

Habitual abortion: See miscarriage.

HCG (human chorionic gonadotropin): A hormone produced by the placenta early in pregnancy and necessary for the maintenance of normal gestation. The blood test called beta subunit of HCG is used to diagnose pregnancy.

Haemophilia: A genetic blood disorder, usually hereditary, characterized by failure of the blood to clot and the occurrence of abnormal bleeding.

Haemorrhage: Profuse bleeding.

Hereditary: Transmitted from generation to generation by way of genes within the chromosomes of the fertilizing sperm and ovum.

Herpes simplex: A virus that can cause blister-like eruptions of mucous membranes such as in the mouth, eyes, and genitals.

High-risk pregnancy: A pregnancy that is at risk for an adverse outcome.

Hormone: A chemical produced and secreted into the blood by the endocrine glands and some organs and that has an effect on other bodily functions, including reproduction.

Human chorionic gonadotropin: *See* HCG.

Hydatidiform mole: *See* molar pregnancy.

Hysterosalpingogram: A procedure in which a dye is introduced into the uterine cavity and coursed through the uterus and fallopian tubes while X-ray pictures are taken to identify scarring, blockages, or other reproductive problems.

Hysteroscopy: A procedure in which a small optical instrument is introduced into the cervix so the doctor can visualize the lining and contour of the uterus, including any fibroid tumours or uterine malformations.

Immunological: That which pertains to the body's natural defences, or immunity, against disease.

Impaired pregnancy: A pregnancy that is abnormal due to environmental, genetic, chromosomal, or unknown causes.

Implantation: The process by which the fertilized egg attaches to the uterine lining.

Incompetent cervix: *See* cervical incompetence.

Incongruent grief: The differing intensity and duration of grief a father and mother may experience.

Incubator: A special enclosed cot for infants in distress that provides controlled temperature and oxygen supply.

Induction of labour: The use of artificial means to stimulate the onset of labour.

Infection: The contamination resulting from harmful bacteria or viruses.

Infertility: The inability to conceive after one year of unprotected intercourse. Repeated consecutive pregnancy losses, without a live birth, may also be referred to as infertility.

Inflammation: A bodily response to irritation or infection involving increased redness, swelling, or pain.

In vitro fertilization (IVF): A procedure in which eggs are surgically removed from a woman and mixed with sperm in a petri dish, after which the fertilized eggs are inserted into a woman's uterus, in an effort to obtain a viable pregnancy.

Karyotype: A photograph of human chromosomes for genetic analysis.

Laminaria sticks: Stems of dried seaweed that absorb moisture, inserted into the cervix to aid dilatation.

Laparoscopy: A procedure performed under general anaesthetic in which an optical instrument, the laparoscope, is inserted through a small incision in the abdominal wall, enabling the doctor to see the fallopian tubes, uterus, and ovaries directly.

Low birth weight: A baby's weight at birth if it is under 2,500 grams (5½ pounds).

Luteal phase defect (LPD): A condition in which too little progesterone is produced following ovulation, affecting the menstrual cycle and the ability to sustain a pregnancy.

Maternal serum alphafetoprotein (MSAFP): A test of the mother's blood that checks for neural tube defects in the unborn baby.

Menstruation (period): The monthly uterine bleeding in which the lining of the womb is expelled from the woman's body if she does not conceive.

Microsurgery: Operations in which special techniques and magnifying instruments are used to correct delicate organs and tissues.

Midwife: A health practitioner, usually a nurse, who specializes in obstetrics.

Miscarriage: A lay term describing early spontaneous loss within the first twenty weeks of pregnancy. The correct medical term is 'abortion,' but many bereaved couples prefer the word 'miscarriage.' There are several types of early miscarriage:

Blighted ovum: An early loss in which the egg was fertilized but no baby developed.

Complete miscarriage: An early loss in which all the products of the conception, including the baby, the sac, and the forming placenta, are expelled from the uterus.

Habitual miscarrier: A woman who has suffered three or more consecutive miscarriages.

Incomplete miscarriage: An early loss in which some products of the pregnancy still remain inside the uterus.

Inevitable miscarriage: An early loss in progress that cannot be stopped.

Missed miscarriage: An early loss in which the baby has died but remains in the uterus, along with the placenta and other elements of conception, without being expelled.

Preclinical pregnancy: An early loss that ends before the woman's next period is due. There are usually no pregnancy symptoms, but a blood test can reveal small amounts of the pregnancy hormone HCG.

Septic miscarriage: An early loss complicated by uterine infection, usually from an incomplete miscarriage.

Spontaneous miscarriage: Any unplanned termination of a pregnancy in the first twenty weeks.

Threatened miscarriage: An incidence in which certain symptoms such as vaginal bleeding or severe cramping occur during pregnancy. The symptoms may stop or may progress to a miscarriage.

Molar pregnancy: The fertilization of an ovum without a nucleus. There is no baby present, and the placenta develops into a non-malignant tumour called a hydatidiform mole.

Mycoplasma (T-strain mycoplasma): A microscopic organism thought to be responsible for pregnancy loss.

Myoma: See fibroid tumour.

Neural tube defect: A birth defect of the brain and/or the spinal cord.

Neonatal: The first twenty-eight days of a baby's life after birth.

Neonatal death: The death of a baby within twenty-eight days of a live birth.

Neonatologist: A paediatrician with specialized training in the care of newborn babies.

Obstetrician: A doctor who specializes in pregnancy and delivery. The field of speciality is called obstetrics.

Oestrogen: The principle female sex hormone that stimulates the reproductive cycle.

Ova: See ovum.

Ovary: The female organs that produce sex hormones and ova, or eggs.

Ovulation: The release of a mature, unfertilized egg from the ovary.

Ovum: The reproductive cell, or egg, of the female. Plural: ova.

Pelvic inflammatory disease (PID): Infection and inflammation of the woman's pelvic organs.

Pelvic or internal examination: A medical examination of the vagina, cervix, uterus, and fallopian tubes.

Perinatal: The period of time from the twentieth week of pregnancy to the twenty-eighth day after birth.

Period: See menstruation.

PID: See pelvic inflammatory disease.

Placenta: The spongy, vascular organ that supplies the baby with maternal blood and nutrients through the umbilical cord.

Placenta praevia: A condition in which the placenta is located over the cervix, creating a risk of haemorrhage during labour and delivery.

Postmature: A baby born after forty-two weeks' gestation.

Preeclampsia: See toxaemia.

Premature: A baby born before thirty-seven weeks' gestation.

Premature labour: The early onset of uterine contractions, generally at least six to eight per hour, accompanied by progressive cervical dilation and effacement between the twentieth and thirty-seventh weeks of pregnancy.

Premature rupture of the membranes (PROM): A break in the amniotic sac, resulting in loss of amniotic fluid, before the onset of labour.

Progesterone: A female hormone important during pregnancy and menstruation.

Prolapsed cord: The expulsion of a portion of the umbilical cord after the membranes have ruptured but before delivery. Pressure on the cord from labour and delivery cuts off the baby's supply of blood and oxygen.

Prostaglandin: A hormone produced by the body that may be administered to induce labour.

Psychotherapist: A health-care professional who treats emotional problems.

Rubella (German measles): A viral disease characterized by headache, fever, rash, and inflammation of the throat. Infection in a pregnant mother can damage the baby.

Saline: A salt solution used for medical procedures.

Scan: A visualization of a woman's reproductive organs achieved by bouncing sound waves into her abdomen. The technique is called sonography or ultrasound.

Special Care Baby Unit (SCBU): A special-care nursery for critically ill newborns, often located in regional medical centres.

Specialist (medical): A doctor who has received advanced training in a specific area of medical care.

Sperm: The male sex cells.

Spina bifida: An abnormality in the development of the spine that can cause severe neurological impairment and paralysis.

Stillbirth: The death of a baby of twenty-four weeks' gestation or more prior to delivery.

Term: Forty weeks' gestation, the normal duration of a pregnancy.

Termination (therapeutic or elective abortion): The ending of a pregnancy by choice.

Toxaemia (preeclampsia): An abnormal condition of late pregnancy characterized by high blood pressure, protein in the urine, and swelling.

Trendelenburg position: The position in which the patient lies on her back with the bed tilted, so that the knees and hips are higher than the head.

Trimester: The term used to define each three-month segment of pregnancy.

T-strain mycoplasma: See mycoplasma.

Ultrasound: See scan.

Umbilical cord: The blood vessels that connect the baby to the placenta.

Uterus (womb): The female reproductive organ that contains the developing baby.

Vagina (birth canal): The organ of the female that forms a passageway between the uterus and the external genitals.

Viability: The ability of an infant to survive outside the uterus.

Virus: A microscopic organism that can cause disease in humans. It differs from bacteria in that it cannot live on its own but must reside inside the cell of another organism.

Womb: See uterus.

INDEX